# The Science of Dignity

# The Science of Dignity

*Measuring Personhood and Well-Being in the United States*

STEVEN HITLIN AND MATTHEW A. ANDERSSON

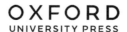

OXFORD
UNIVERSITY PRESS

# OXFORD
## UNIVERSITY PRESS

Published in the United States of America by Oxford University Press
198 Madison Avenue, New York, NY 10016, United States of America.

Library of Congress Cataloging-in-Publication Data
Names: Hitlin, Steven, Andersson, Matthew A., editors.
Title: The science of dignity: measuring personhood and well-being in the United States /
Steven Hitlin, Matthew A. Andersson.
Description: New York, NY : Oxford University Press, [2023] |
Includes bibliographical references and index. |
Identifiers: LCCN 2023007364 (print) | LCCN 2023007365 (ebook) |
ISBN 9780197743867 (hardback) | ISBN 9780197743881 (epub) |
ISBN 9780197743898
Subjects: LCSH: Social psychology—United States. | Dignity.
Classification: LCC HM1033 .S258 2023 (print) | LCC HM1033 (ebook) |
DDC 302—dc23/eng/20230406
LC record available at https://lccn.loc.gov/2023007364
LC ebook record available at https://lccn.loc.gov/2023007365

DOI: 10.1093/oso/9780197743867.001.0001

Printed by Sheridan Books, Inc., United States of America

# Contents

Contents

# Acknowledgments

We have consolidated this project over many years. Earlier, smaller incarnations of it have appeared in our conversations, handbook chapters, and article drafts. To see our approach to dignity come to life in book form is both a delight and an honor. We have separate parties to thank:

Hitlin: This project has been academically invigorating over the past almost decade, starting with a quirky idea that Matt Andersson had in response to an invitation for us to write a book chapter, and working a few articles and chapters into this manuscript. Thanks to Matt for unflagging energy, idea generation, and a passion for making tables and running quantitative analyses that you would have to see to believe.

Thanks to all the various friends, family members, and colleagues and others who make life worth living and hold a special place in my life. During the creation of this book, I've also cocreated three boys who have added an entire new dimension to my life. I'm grateful to Ellen, Jones, Sam, and Ian—and our dog, Greta, as the boys would remind me to mention.

Andersson: The importance of bringing more dignity to more people by getting the word out through science helped me stay focused and positive—and occasionally even downright happy about the project. Thank you to Steve Hitlin for maintaining the vision and ambition for us over the years, and for encouraging population health arguments that do not typically reside near morality or social theory.

Thank you to my family and friends for your curiosity and encouragement about the project. Thanks especially to my mother, Shari Porte, for her unflagging love, optimism, and insight; to my father, Lars Andersson, for living with resilience and curiosity; and to my brother, Elliott Andersson, for being the human being who is most similar to me. Thank you to Paul Froese for reading an early draft of the book's initial chapters and for providing great kernels of insight for revising them; to Chris Pieper for validating some of my ideas and adding to parts of them; and to stef shuster for their enlightening perspective and useful comments. Thanks to Matt Lee for orienting me to dignity as a possible public health concern, to Shai Dromi and Laura Upenieks for their careful feedback earlier on, to Leah Keesee for talking about potential ways of defining dignity, to Monica O'Desky for asking how the book was going and talking with me about its progress, to Pinewood Coffee Bar for their kind and inspiring atmosphere teeming with music, and to Catherine Ballas for likening social interaction to dance and for her points about shame and vulnerability.

We thank a few audiences for providing great and insightful feedback on content for this book, including The University of Iowa College of Law and the Harvard University Culture Workshop in 2022, the Baylor University Human Flourishing Brownbag in 2021, Duke University's Kenan Ethics Institute in 2018, and fellow sociologists in New York City in 2019 (at the annual meeting of the American Sociological Association).

Thank you to the Baylor University Department of Sociology, and to Paul Froese in particular, for enthusiastically supporting my career and for investing in the 2017 and 2021 Gallup Values and Beliefs of the American Public survey.

# Introduction

## More Than a Feeling

### Dignity and Health Inequalities in America

### Thinking about Dignity: Where the Social Meets the Personal

In the twenty-first century, each life in a democratic society is considered sacred, at least abstractly. Yet, from calls for social justice, to worker layoffs and strikes, to conversations about the effects of cyberbullying and cancel culture, it has become essentially impossible for a person in America to avoid thinking about their social relationships—and how those relationships might be different or better.

The concept of dignity appears pivotal to many of these recent discussions. For instance, lawyers for George Floyd's family stated: "Tens of thousands of Americans struggle with self-medication and opioid abuse and are treated with dignity, respect and support, not brutality."[1] Years earlier, the archbishop emeritus Desmond Tutu remarked, "We seem somehow to have forgotten that all beings are equal in dignity, the tenet in the first article of the Universal Declaration of Human Rights."[2]

Dignity exists and forms at the intersection of self and society, as societies create and recognize individuals and vice versa. Social relationships reflect or defy cultural understandings. Dignity could be lost by how one is treated while alive—or in one's tragic death. If one's life does not matter to others, dignity might exist only as a legal or religious abstraction. A cultural logic of "what matters" or "mattering" or "people mattering"—co-opted by corporate mission statements and social movements alike—carries the sobering, basic implication that a person's or group's dignity might be held in question.

---

[1] "George Floyd's Girlfriend Says Opioid Addiction Was a Struggle They Shared," *New York Times*, April 1, 2021.
[2] Tutu is quoted in Foreword of *Dignity* by Donna Hicks.

*The Science of Dignity*. Steven Hitlin and Matthew A. Andersson, Oxford University Press.

Dignity is a difficult-to-define term, one that is leveraged to win arguments. Appeals to dignity anchor calls for social change while reflecting a perceived "fair" relationship between individuals and societies. To support dignity is to be on the side of goodness, even as the term is employed by all sides in social and political debates. Appeals to dignity, whether protecting the right to safety from hateful or lethal violence, the right to bear arms, or the right to choose one's reproductive options, echo throughout society and suggest it is contested rather than always assumed. Where many favor health promotion, others point to "identity politics."[3]

Clearly, dignity and morality are deeply intertwined (Lamont 2000). Even as moralities are diverse, dignity carries a sense of universal value. In fact, given how it typically foregrounds the sanctity of individual life, dignity could help constitute a unifying morality in pluralistic, democratic societies such as the United States (Dworkin 2006; Lamont 2019; Neal 2014). Charles Taylor (1991) suggests that this "concept of dignity is the only one compatible with a democratic society" (46). In a pluralistic society, we are entrusted with the capacity to tolerate and learn from others deemed unlike ourselves (Gelfand et al. 2011).

In this book, we make the original argument that dignity in its own right—as a concept—has important consequences for health and well-being. In America and elsewhere, people are bound to disagree about the specifics of how to achieve dignity. Despite this, we find that dignity is profoundly affected by one's social roles and stresses, and by the economic, psychological, and social resources that one possesses. Individuals in more advantaged social positions—marked by greater resources and fewer sources of chronic or harmful stress—report the highest levels of dignity. *Because dignity associates so strongly with numerous indicators of health and well-being, we make the case that dignity is a public health concern that has been overlooked for too long, because we have not been able to agree on what it means.*

Like individuals deeming themselves as "happy" or as leading a "meaningful life," allowing individuals to interpret "dignity" for themselves—as individual, moral subjects—helps to circumvent philosophical, theoretical,

---

[3] An irony is that liberatory or movement-based origins of this phrase have become considerably obscured by restrictive or discriminatory uses, as is the case here: "Every time this article is revised, it is tempting to write that 'identity politics' is an outmoded term, over-determined by its critics and part of a reductive political lexicon on both the Marxist left and the neoconservative right." Entry on "Identity Politics," Stanford Encyclopedia of Philosophy, substantive revision July 11, 2020.

and legal debates about dignity's "true" meaning. We contend that a subjective, public-based approach to measuring dignity is overdue, and that it will pay considerable dividends in moving forward a science of dignity: who thinks they have it, how and why it matters, and what we can do about it to improve societies and individual lives and the harmful health inequality we see in America.

To measure how dignity matters in America, we make novel use of a pair of national datasets that we collected in cooperation with Gallup and the Department of Sociology at Baylor University in spring 2017 and again in spring 2021. Using these data, we document perceptions of dignity among individuals in America before and during the Covid-19 pandemic. By describing and tracking the social distribution of dignity in terms of whether individuals from differing social backgrounds view their own lives as dignified, we gain insight into who thinks they have dignity and the potential consequences of these dignity perceptions. We uncover how dignity associates with demographics, health, social networks, and other aspects of life in a way that begins to clarify what dignity means to the people who live it out—and, with this, what possible effects dignity as a social concept might have on diverse American lives.

Is dignity something more than treating others with respect and expecting respect in turn? If so, what makes it different? And when ideas of morality differ so much in today's polarized political climate, can dignity hope to mean something more than just the individual freedom to ignore or disagree?

We make the case that studying dignity helps promote a person-centered approach to the study of health inequalities in America. If we could measure dignity, we might be able to identify factors associated with its improvement. The stakes have never been higher. Breaking from an overly individualistic point of view and teaching solidarity with and recognition of others might be one key basis of how social scientists can serve the world today. Policymakers and politicians might even work alongside scientists to help promote new ways of finding value and worth despite our many differences.[4]

---

[4] These aspirational goals for social scientists and politicians are sourced from Michèle Lamont's recent public lecture, "Breaking the Wall to Universal Dignity," delivered in December 2022.

## A Science of Dignity: "If We Cannot Measure It, How Will We Know We're Achieving It?"

In a comment submitted to *The Lancet*, one of the most prominent and oldest medical journals in the world, the social epidemiologist Sir Michael Marmot (2004) said, "If we cannot define dignity precisely, we will have trouble measuring it. If we cannot measure it, how will we know we are achieving it?"

Marmot essentially suggests that stalemates about dignity's definition have stalled the development of data collection on dignity. In this book, we offer an approach to measuring dignity that acknowledges dignity's complexity without dismissing it. We argue and show that by asking people whether they have dignity, and by looking at the social conditions of their lives, we might learn more about what dignity *actually* is—not what we might *assume* it is.

By showing how dignity is patterned in America, we hope to change our social understandings of dignity. These changed social understandings, in turn, might lead us to imagine and perhaps even act on better futures, both individually and collectively. In this way, a science of dignity could "serve as conceptual resources for an entire culture" (Callero 2003, 127).

## Subjective Dignity as a Public Health Concern

We begin with a quick overview of the national Gallup survey we use to capture perceptions of dignity in America. In collaboration with Gallup, we employed three dignity survey items in 2017 and again in 2021 (Figure I.1).

GALLUP

| Please rate the extent to which you agree or disagree with the following statements. ••• | Strongly disagree ▼ | Disagree ▼ | Agree ▼ | Stronly agree ▼ | Undecided ▼ |
|---|---|---|---|---|---|
| g.  I feel that my life lacks dignity. | ☐ | ☐ | ☐ | ☐ | ☐ |
| h.  People generally treat me with dignity. | ☐ | ☐ | ☐ | ☐ | ☐ |
| i.  I determine my own dignity. | ☐ | ☐ | ☐ | ☐ | ☐ |

**Figure I.1** Survey Items on Subjective Perceptions of Dignity, 2017 and 2021 Values and Beliefs of the American Public Survey

**"I feel that my life lacks dignity"** captures an overall assessment of dignity in and about one's life. **"People generally treat me with dignity"** taps into dignity's interpersonal and relational dimensions. **"I determine my own dignity"** was designed to capture a fundamental relationship between dignity and autonomy, in terms of how individuals can actively maintain dignity through how they exert control over their own lives or choose to relate to the situations they encounter.

These three items are not meant to offer a complete measurement of dignity. However, they do reflect dignity's multiple dimensions. Most importantly, we ask about "dignity" without invoking predetermined ideas about what, exactly, this term might mean to different individuals in varying social situations.

By using our innovative survey approach, we find that dignity represents a public health issue. Individuals who report low levels of dignity—or what we call *dignity threat*—are 3.7 times more likely to be unhappy, and over twice as likely to be in lower health or feel depressed, compared to those with moderate to high levels of dignity. Individuals with threatened dignity levels also are significantly more likely to feel angry or have difficulty sleeping (Figure I.2).

DIGNITY THREAT as a Public Health Issue

Unhappy    3.7x
Depressed    2.3x
Angry    1.7x
Difficulty Sleeping  1.4x
--------------------------------------
Fair/Poor Health  2.4x

**Figure I.2** Increased Prevalence of Health Issues with Dignity Threat

Note: Individuals with low or threatened levels of dignity are compared to individuals with moderate to high levels of dignity. 1.0× represents no difference in health, while 2.0× (3.0×) means that a health problem is twice (or three times) as common among those with threatened dignity.

A full 21.5% of Americans in spring 2021 reported that their dignity was under threat. This percentage figure reflects an increase of over 50% relative to levels of dignity threat seen in the 2017 Gallup survey (Figure I.3).

**Gallup** Values and Beliefs of the American Public Survey
(Given in all 50 U.S. States & District of Columbia, 2017 and 2021)

*any dignity threat*   (Based on All Items)
2021                                          2017

**21.5%** of National Sample      14.1%
(↑52% from 2017)

Item-Specific Breakdowns

"I feel that my life lacks dignity."
□ Strongly Agree (5.6%, ↑273% vs. 2017)      □ Agree (7.5%, ↑34% vs. 2017)

"People generally treat me with dignity."
□ Strongly Disagree (2.2%, ↑100% vs. 2017)   □ Disagree (5.8%, ↑35% vs. 2017)

"I determine my own dignity."
□ Strongly Disagree (2.7%, ↑21% vs. 2017)     □ Disagree (3.6%, ↑33% vs. 2017)

**Figure I.3**  Tracking Dignity Threat from 2017 to 2021 Based on National Gallup Survey Data

*Note.* Survey item response categories corresponding to perceived dignity threat are shown.

## Defining Dignity: The Stakes Are High

The sociologist Georg Simmel noted that when we see another person, we see them as if through a veil, in terms of who they are to us socially, which is an incomplete way of viewing an individual compared with how they see themselves. People are to us what they mean to us, and what they mean to us is greatly determined by social categories, resources, and relationships. "I can believe in all that has been lost in translation," writes the poet James Richardson, "though all works, all acts, all languages are already translation." Social translation can lead to affiliation or to violence—individuals cannot live without their societies, and sometimes cannot live with them either.

Many if not most people who live in America could be lacking in dignity if dignity is considered as social status or honor; only so many people become wealthy or famous. However, people also develop ways of thinking and talking about their lives that support a sense of being dignified even despite objective hardship, social marginalization, or not subscribing to dominant cultural views. To put it simply: people *encounter* all manner of hardship, and they *counter* those hardships with their autonomy or how they matter to others they care about. No person—high-status or low-status—is immune from harm to their dignity. Magnitudes, causes, and consequences of dignity violations differ profoundly, however, depending on one's position in society.

So, how should we define dignity? And who gets to define it? These questions are particularly timely in view of what George Packer in *The Atlantic* magazine recently labeled Four Americas: Free America, Real America, Smart America, and Just America.[5] Free America has its modern counterparts in Republicanism and libertarianism; Real America in working-class virtues and struggles; Smart America in cosmopolitanism, higher education, and meritocratic strife; and Just America in a justice-centered critique of meritocracy revealing its origins and operations steeped in—soaked in—colonialism and wealth. Packer, like many scholars, has characterized various strands in America's grand narrative that compete within individual minds and the collective imagination alike.

Nowadays, when Gerard Baker writes in the *Wall Street Journal* that he sees in critical race theory (CRT) "the opposite of education" and casts CRT as "un-American," this speaks again to Packer's typology of America narratives; one can just as easily cast CRT as quintessentially American—that is, an overdue illumination of how to extend dignity to Black Americans.[6] The Northwestern psychologist Dan McAdams (2013a, 2013b) sees contamination and adversity in America's history as much as he sees possibilities of resilience and progress, and he notes how countless life stories in America intertwine these twin, tragic themes.

Vaccine debates have generated polarizing punchlines such as "[a] bullet for the country but not a needle for a neighbor," yet another instantiation of America's internal narrative fault lines. What it means and looks like to care is fundamental to dignity. If Alabama governor Kay Ivey can increase vaccination rates by pointing out how vaccine development and Operation Warp Speed are related, this reveals some of the different ways Americans can be moved to care.[7]

In the wake of George Floyd's murder, some commentators noted the price tags of property destruction, and this led to a dialogue about how to protect priceless lives. Human lives are priceless, and yet society is not currently structured in a way that prices lives equally. Life expectancies differ dramatically by US state, by race, and by social class; the Harvard epidemiologist David Williams notes how zip or postal code supersedes genetic code

[5] "How America Fractured into Four Parts," *The Atlantic*, July/August 2021.
[6] "Critical Race Theory Is the Opposite of Education," *Wall Street Journal*, June 21, 2021.
[7] Kay Ivey, "Opinion: The Trump Administration Gave Us the Best Weapons against Covid-19. We Should Use Them," *Washington Post*, July 27, 2021.

in predicting a healthy life, indeed translating to fewer *decades* of life for extremely disadvantaged individuals.[8]

Upon looking around at different forms of inequality in American society, the notion of "dignity" might understandably ring hollow. As societies seem to disintegrate, is dignity an ideal, a reality, both, or neither? Tellingly, it is hard to define dignity without using the word itself. Dignity might elude a precise or singular definition because, in practice, it should: perhaps it refers to a *set* of practical realities.[9]

"Living with dignity" might involve being dignified and treated with dignity; dying unjustly or not dying a good death raises the issue of "dying with dignity."[10] History, technology, or circumstance may change our interpretation of whether a life was lived in vain, leading to changing assessments of that death's dignity on behalf of the dead. Treatment of a body after death raises a whole separate set of issues regarding dignity. To witness this fact, one need only look to coroners working across Kyiv in the aftermath of the Russian invasion: "I'm used to seeing horrible things done to bodies," one coroner said. "But I was very shocked to see such horrible treatment of the deceased by the Russians. How can someone shoot a person and then run over the body?"[11]

## Building a Sociological Foundation for a Science of Dignity

Social life is multifaceted; dignity's relatedly puzzling nature is to be expected. As we contend in this book, declaring dignity "useless" simply because it seems too complicated is a form of intellectual evasion. Yet, developing a science of a slippery term runs into real risks of producing too many definitions or complicating what is already viewed to be of fundamental importance in some religious, legal, humanitarian, or political circles. We cannot ignore dignity's complexity, but we cannot ossify this term either. Rather than

---

[8] Risa Lavizzo-Mourey and David Williams, "Being Black Is Bad for Your Health," *US News and World Report*, April 14, 2016.

[9] The same might be said for the notions of situated personhood or human agency more generally, conceptualizations of social individuality that likewise carry historical and material contingencies (see, e.g., Bourdieu 1990; Emirbayer and Mische 1998; Granovetter 1985; Hitlin and Elder 2007; Joas 1996; Sewell 1992).

[10] For a great, contextualized treatment of social considerations surrounding death, see Mara Buchbinder's (2021) *Scripting Death*.

[11] "One Body at a Time, a Kyiv Coroner Documents Ukraine's Death Toll," *Washington Post*, April 20, 2022.

overriding existing, important discussions of dignity, we are trying to illuminate them further by using a new survey methodology.

Dignity offers a valuable opportunity to illuminate the moral, social person. Somewhat like dignity, love (Swidler 2001) might be defined in terms of commitment or self-growth, or its neurobiological correlates or the emotions or sensations it produces, but it means something very different to each person, even as its consequences or value may be universally accepted.

In fact, it might be more useful to think of "dignities" or social conceptions of dignity as a starting basis of an empirical science of dignity, rather than any all-purpose conception. The sociologist Allison Pugh (2012, p. 30) recommends a similar approach: "What if we thought about dignity instead as a social construct, something that refers to our capacity to stand as fully recognized participants in our social world, that derives its very meaning from its social context?" Today, dignity spans multiple levels of social reality. Appeals to dignity as an explanative factor range from its being a "hidden" cultural factor underlying robust national development (Hojman and Miranda 2018) to an intrapsychic buffer against personal experiences of marginalization within unequal, deeply classed and racialized societies (Bonilla-Silva 2010; Lamont 2017; Wilkerson 2020).

Dignity is a multilevel, moral belief system that is operative at both the individual and collective levels.[12] At the individual level, it is a tool for understanding and justifying one's actions and one's self. Meanwhile, it provides guides for offering tact to others and successful social interaction in homes, neighborhoods, workplaces, schools, and other community settings. At the collective or societal level, it provides visions of humanity and equality that are useful for framing debates and realizing rights within political discourse.

How individuals and societies ought to relate starts with the very nature of what it means to be a person. The eminent psychologist Susan Fiske (2004) summarizes a century of psychological research by highlighting five fundamental human motives in social life: belonging, understanding, controlling, self-enhancement, and trust. We suggest that dignity, because it refers to personhood, might integrate people's subjective senses of how these multiple needs are being met: whether individuals feel like they belong and are meaningfully understood, are in some control of their own lives, can present a positive image to those around them, and trust others and the larger world. Personhood can and should be studied at the confluence of these many

---

[12] Thank you to Paul Froese for this excellent and useful conceptualization.

motivations and the diverse situations that individuals experience daily and in the long run. Whether individuals feel dignified as people is likely to be correspondingly complicated.

Craig Calhoun (1991) noted how sociology has become "unmusical" when it comes to documenting how people experience their lives, circumstances, and other people. There are tens of thousands of papers and books and studies to wade through in sociology and social science more generally. The urge for generalization in some corners of social science (e.g., Healy 2017) can come at the cost of understanding lived experience (e.g., Blumer 1969). In this book, we want to understand social processes while incorporating subjective notions of individual lives (e.g., Hitlin 2008). By doing so, we can encounter universal value through our subjective experience of it: "There must be something in man that gives rise to this feeling that his nature is dual, a feeling that men in all known civilizations have experienced," Emile Durkheim once wrote.[13]

Privilege has been defined as relative freedom from different struggles or oppressions within society, while marginalization represents a relative absence of such advantages, as well as stigmatization or even persecution. As Roxane Gay (2014) usefully observed, not being wholly privileged or wholly marginalized does not abrogate one of the responsibility to be aware of one's intersectional existence, since everyone has multiple statuses and therefore lives across multiple hierarchies of status or value all at once. A realistic approach to individuality could involve affirming the self while also acknowledging historical and social advantage that has created or enabled aspects of one's present social situation (Phillips and Lowery 2015). And while individuals might debate the very bases of privileges or marginalization, as is common on Twitter or on cable news networks, sociologists are equipped with national data on individual resources, demographic background, and levels of health and well-being in a way that can shed urgently needed light on the life-or-death meanings of these social categories.

By making individuals the subject of their own dignity, we stand to gain more knowledge about how dignity works. A problem with using predetermined definitions of dignity is that dignity is profoundly personal, even among those who share similar events or social groupings. Despite a popular view that everyone is unique and perhaps relatedly that dignity is therefore unquantifiable,

[13] "The Dualism of Human Nature and Its Social Conditions" [Le Dualisme de la Nature Humaine et ses Conditions Sociales], *Revue Philosophique*, February 1916.

we find in this book that levels and predictors of dignity are still shaped in patterned ways by resources, locations, and identities: age, education, gender, geography, political ideology, religiosity, and so forth. Meanwhile, crucially, there also is a great deal of variation within these categories, based in personal biographies that are woven together at the phenomenological intersection of thought, experience, and personality.

## Numbed by Numbers: Does a Science of Dignity Perpetuate or Help the Problem?

From time to emails to money to profits, numbers are everywhere in everyday life. Many of us are time-crazed—measuring ourselves against a tantalizing finish line of so-called Inbox Zero. Careerism follows from cultural understandings of the ideal worker, who is always available or always on call. The ideal worker, in turn, is anchored in the core belief that with hard work, all is possible (Frye 2019; Mijs 2018).

As the sociologist Philip Hodgkiss (2018) points out, Kant's "implicit universalism" of dignity-within-and-for-all becomes problematic within a capitalist society that lives or dies by numbers. Modern capitalism emphasizes acts and logics of quantification (Chun and Sauder 2022), such as thinking about workers in terms of the maximization of profits or efficiencies. Ever since Max Weber outlined how this process is socially shaped, the direction of more rationality, bureaucracy, and institutionalization only ratchets upward:[14] de-quantification rarely happens due to how quantification is a logic that becomes embedded in organizational operations through structure, practices, power, and culture (Chun and Sauder 2022; Sauder and Espeland 2009). Quantification can also be inadvertently worsened through calls for accountability, transparency, or efficiency across law, industry, medicine, or education (Espeland and Sauder 2007).

In a world that often puts a price on you, can you separate your own self-worth from your wage, salary, or wealth? Some might think so, but apparently even millionaires say they need two to three times their current wealth to be perfectly happy,[15] and Matthew Killingsworth (2021) found using over

---

[14] This does not mean that people become more rational or that societies make decisions more efficiently. Instead, systems designed for efficiency spread, trapping us in Weber's notorious "iron cage."

[15] See survey results reported in "Why Aren't Rich People Happy with the Money They Have?," *The Atlantic*, December 4, 2018.

one million experience-sampling data points that more money is associated with greater life satisfaction even into the six figures.

Dignity is distinct from happiness or life satisfaction, but, as we just saw, unhappy people are more than three times as likely to report a lack of dignity to their lives. As Edgar Cabanas and Eva Illouz (2019) noted, there is social danger in implying that happiness is a choice; if happiness and indignity are intertwined, then much of happiness—and much of dignity—might rest in how society treats us. The social psychologist Sonja Lyubomirsky has made this very argument, by carving up the happiness pie into circumstances, choices, and genetics, allotting a generous portion to circumstances based on hundreds of research studies.

Based on the copious self-help literature, one might think circumstances cannot prevent happiness if you just try hard enough, but if one is realistic, then plenty of circumstances set limits on happiness. Even if someone is not happy, they can benefit from a sense of control, mattering to others, a sense of purpose in life, or numerous other psychological, economic, and social resources that we cover in this book when mapping out dignity levels in Americans' lives.

A fundamental tension in modern life—and, perhaps not coincidentally, in the interdisciplinary literature on dignity—consists in the paradoxical reality of human lives being both intrinsically priceless and socially priced. Scholars often quote Immanuel Kant's distinction between price and dignity: that which has dignity, such as human life, is invaluable or cannot have a price. Yet, modern insurance firms, legal settlements, and other institutions justify their existence through finding socially convincing ways of pricing the priceless.[16] Zelizer (1979) traces how, for example, life insurance went from a macabre business proposition toward a morally righteous thing to purchase "for your family."

We are numbed by numbers in today's numeric society. Quantification can impede dignity, but quantifying levels of dignity, through a scientific approach to dignity contained in this book, might help to begin to restore dignity in a way that means something more than numbers. *By measuring levels*

[16] Kant reserved dignity for morality and viewed human life as dignified only insofar as it is moral. We return to this theme in later chapters. Essentially, we argue that a broader interpretation of morality in line with Adam Smith's equation of the social with the moral might be what many scholars have in mind when appropriating Kant on dignity and would resolve a lot of inherent contradictions in the term enough to let us deploy it in social science.

*of dignity in America, we can learn more about how individuals think about dignity, what might actually shape it, and what dignity's effects might be.*

What are some potential drawbacks of enumerating and comparing dignity levels? Quantitative rankings of dignity across different individuals or groups in society might have the appearance of denying the *absolute* subjective reality of suffering by construing it in *relative* terms, to paraphrase the essayist Zadie Smith (2020). For instance, if an individual perceives twice the level of dignity in their life than another individual does, that could be because of absolute differences in life conditions or due to subjective differences in how individuals think about those conditions. More likely, it is some combination of both. One cannot numerically reason one's way to human dignity—it simply *is*—just as one cannot reason, in any purely logical sense, one's way to a particular valuation of human life.

## Overviewing This Book

The first chapters of this book discuss what many minds across the centuries have thought about dignity.[17] We overview how dignity as a popular concept is present in multiple intellectual and professional circles—religion, moral philosophy, and social theory, and then constitutional and human rights law—and how it has diffused outward to the public. We begin within intellectual or academic backgrounds because dignity is an element of public culture that is sourced from these institutional origins (Lizardo 2017; Swidler 2001). That is, individuals learn about what dignity might mean by encountering and interpreting these cultural, legal, academic, and popular definitions that diffuse outward from social institutions and by "trying them out" within their own lives.

This book has two distinct sections. The first section, contained in Chapters 1 through 4, provides an overview on leading perspectives on and theories about dignity. The second section, which encompasses Chapters 5 through 10, contains our approach to measuring subjective dignity and how it matters in America.

---

[17] Those seeking a more purely intellectual genealogy of the concept would be better served by brilliantly written titles such as Michael Rosen's (2012) *Dignity* or Philip Hodgkiss' (2018) *Social Thought and Rival Claims to the Moral Ideal of Dignity.*

## Chapter 1: A Wide-Ranging Tour of Perspectives on Dignity

We provide an overview of leading accounts and definitions of dignity, sourced from philosophy, human rights law, and the social and medical sciences. How the public thinks about dignity has diffused from these social institutions. We discuss how dignity often is understood against proposed synonyms such as autonomy or respect, or in the context of phrasal uses (such as "dying with dignity" or "beneath one's dignity").

Rather than throwing up our hands at this complexity, we find it is far more useful to think of dignity as a practical, situational experience rather than a formally defined entity. We offer a sociological critique of Kantian approaches to dignity that focus on rationality or autonomy in generalized terms. With this, we provide an overview of current approaches to dignity in sociology, which measure it in terms of power or hierarchy, especially at work, and in terms of how individuals cope with or resist mistreatment or unfairness.

## Chapter 2: Seeing Circles: Dignity as a Public Health Issue

To begin establishing dignity as a public health issue, we explore suicide as a social problem. We then discuss population health in twin, contrasting ways: average health across a population and variation in health by different social circles. Rising tides do not lift all boats, and individuals inhabit multiple social circles that shape their dignity, rather than a so-called average life. Specific murders or injustices teach us about society's ongoing conflicts. To gain finer resolution on social injustice, we turn to the idea of status characteristics, which are attachments of social value to social categories: gender, class, race, age, ability, and other demographic characteristics. Given this hierarchical backdrop, we define the relationship between dignity and population health as one of social endurance: preserving and defining individuality against the social violence that group-based inequalities imply.

## Chapter 3: Beyond Reason: Finding Dignity in Social Relations

We define dignity as a public health issue in terms of mattering and relating to others. By emphasizing how social chaos unravels social relationships, we show how care acts as a motivation that maintains and sustains dignity. Dignity rests in the creative and emotional nature of social interaction. Despite idealistic arguments about dignity as moral calculation, rationality without emotion is not rationality at all. Moreover, because social interactions are transactional—individuals are constituted by and through social interaction—people become ends or reasons for themselves and for others, and morality orients around people and their moments rather than principles and their abstractions. Thus, dignity is oriented around people and the moralities that they, in turn, orient.

## Chapter 4: American Capitalism and Its Multifaceted Links to Dignity

Our macro perspective on dignity and public health positions people within American capitalism. We observe indignity across the American class structure, whether in terms of ritualistic overwork among the professional classes or in terms of precarity or being shut out of institutions among the working classes. We trace these pervasive indignities to how capitalism uneasily juxtaposes—and thrives on the distressing tension between—quantification and efficiency on the one hand and individualism and equity on the other hand. More specifically, we locate the indignity of capitalism in the systemic, predictable way that capitalism entwines and operates on the status characteristics we discussed earlier. That is, classism, racism, sexism, ableism, and ageism all are implicit or plainly visible in how capitalism assigns and quantifies worth. We draw concrete illustrations from literatures on college inequality, pandemic inequality, ideal worker inequality, and privatization of risk to illustrate how this works.

## Chapter 5: Measuring Dignity Subjectively: Methodology for 2017 and 2021 Gallup Data

We outline our measurement strategy for subjective dignity and its justification. Subjective dignity is measured, as introduced above, through whether people think they have dignity in their own lives. By comparing dignity to the gold standard measure of self-rated health—one of the most important measures across the social sciences—we can learn what to expect from a comprehensive, subjective measure. Just as self-rated health is predicted by but not reducible to objective health information such as symptoms or conditions, we expect that dignity should overlap somewhat with important social and moral processes such as respect, discrimination, and mattering, as well as objective social class or demographic differences, while not being reducible to any one of these predictors. We give background information on the dignity survey items and subjective dignity scale construction, and we address key strengths and limitations of our subjective dignity measurement approach from the standpoints of quantification of people and conducting cross-sectional survey research into health.

## Chapter 6: Dignity as an Efficient Indicator of Social and Moral Integration

We provide an overview of survey response patterns for subjective dignity from 2017 to 2021. Rates of "dignity threat" increased in the American population by about 50%. Next, we test whether dignity is linked to relevant measures of social and moral functioning. Dignity bears expected associations with respect from others and specific people such as employers and doctors, and it also varies strongly with perceived discrimination. While dignity bears some association with general or specific moral principles such as accountability to others or to God or one's happiness, the links are not particularly strong, consistent with the fact that dignity perceptions do not tether to any one moral code in America. Mastery, or a sense of control over this life, and mattering to others and perceiving meaning in life constitute what we call the "three Ms" when it comes to understanding a large portion of the variation in dignity.

## Chapter 7: Is a Dignified Life a Healthier Life?

We find that individuals who report subjective dignity also report better past, current, and predicted health and lesser frequency of depressive symptoms. These associations hold across a variety of demographic backgrounds and rival in size those linked to income and social status. Meanwhile, individuals experiencing dignity threat are much more likely to report a variety of health issues. An instrumental variable analysis provides support for the proposition that dignity leads to better health. Dignity relates to better health net of mastery, life meaning, and mattering to others. In fact, it is most strongly linked to general health when these other resources are lacking, suggesting its unique role in promoting well-being among those who are structurally or extremely disadvantaged.

## Chapter 8: A Resource-Based Framework for Analyzing Levels of Dignity

We develop and test a framework that analyzes dignity variation in terms of differences in economic, psychological, and social resources possessed by individuals. As individuals accumulate more of these resources, they also report higher levels of subjective dignity. At the same time, particular resources vary considerably in their degree of overlap with dignity, and the resource model shows varying degrees of fit across different demographic groups. Meanwhile, we document that a four-year college degree is a powerful social determinant of numerous resource differences. Finally, we lend complexity to the nature of social connectedness, by allowing it to take digital and in-person forms. We find that individuals who integrate digital and in-person connectedness show the highest levels of subjective dignity.

## Chapter 9: Inequality and Stress: Charting Dignity during Social Adversity

Social categorizations such as race, sex, age, and class imply much more than differences in resources. They also generate varying degrees of social stress. We break out declines in subjective dignity from 2017 to 2021 for numerous demographic groups. Generally, we find that overall losses in dignity across the pandemic have been greater for minoritized and vulnerable groups, with some exceptions. Then, we document declines in dignity linked to specific stressors, such as missing house or rent payments, increasing debt, going hungry, experiencing serious conflict at home, and being unable to afford health care. We show how Blacks, Hispanics, women, and sexual/gender minorities are disproportionately likely to experience these stressors. Additionally, we find that physically disabled individuals lost dignity at three times the rate of nondisabled individuals from 2017 and 2021, and we analyze this steep loss in terms of health, work, financial, and network difficulties that disability entails.

## Chapter 10: One Polarized Nation: Dignity across Political Ideologies

Separating dignity losses by political ideology, we find that liberals lost more dignity from 2017 to 2021 than conservatives or moderates. Across these ideological lines, the importance of respect to dignity is consistently emphasized, and dignity's relationship to a variety of health issues is quite consistent as well. The resource model of dignity finds considerable support across ideology as well, but this support varies depending on year and ideology. Particular psychological, economic, and social resources also show divergent associations with dignity across ideology. What unites political parties is that they all report polarization. Thus, we conclude the chapter by looking at how polarization relates to subjective dignity levels. Increased polarization, measured in terms of feeling threatened by a greater number of groups in society, is linked to indignity in the American population.

# 1

# A Wide-Ranging Tour of Perspectives on Dignity

In "The Greatest Love of All," Whitney Houston sang that dignity belongs to her and cannot be taken away by anyone. Dignity seems given or inviolable—even as we see, label, and recognize its violation.

Barack Obama would not need to say "human dignity cannot be denied" if dignity was undeniable. Dignity may be a birthright, but in practice it is socially fragile. As noted by Michèle Lamont (2018), a sociologist at Harvard University who has been writing on dignity for decades, lower-status groups in society develop ways of gleaning recognition and worth despite their more frequent exposure to adversities. Despite these coping efforts, society's hierarchy still tends to perpetuate what Lamont calls "recognition gaps" according to social categories such as gender, race, class, or age, for example.

Dignity is an encompassing term, allowing its power to anchor legal systems (Düwell et al., 2014). After World War II, Eleanor Roosevelt helped to draft the Universal Declaration of Human Rights that declared humans "born free and equal in dignity and rights." This text has influenced a range of subsequent national constitutions and modern legal systems, codifying equal worth and equal rights in a world where war and genocide have threatened their existence (Düwell et al. 2014; Weinrib 2016). Meanwhile, modern constitutional democracies speak of individuals as means rather than as ends (Dworkin 2006; Habermas 2010). Dignity has been positioned within intergroup relations, as a sense of—and quest for—"mutual respect across the boundaries of inequality" (Sennett 2003, 99).

Dignity's absence could be considered a public health crisis, if only we could measure exactly what it is that we are talking about. Humiliation, abuse, violence, poverty, and discrimination are profound adversities thought to diminish dignity, and yet dignity seems to mean much more than the absence of suffering or the presence of individual resilience (Sanchez, Lamont, and Zilberstein 2022).

*The Science of Dignity.* Steven Hitlin and Matthew A. Andersson, Oxford University Press.
© Oxford University Press 2023. DOI: 10.1093/oso/9780197743867.003.0002

Dignity is fundamentally cultural, not defined strictly by material conditions or counting one's adversities. That is, it stems from collectively shared meanings, resources, or norms within societies, social groups, and individual lives (Lamont et al. 2016). While human rights violations and constitutional and criminal law offer valuable points of departure for understanding what dignity is, dignity must ultimately be understood on a practical, broader basis if it is to have full scientific value.

In this chapter, we discuss concepts related to dignity, as well as differing senses in which "dignity" has been used by a variety of noted personalities—not just scholars and researchers. Our overall aim in the coming pages is to lay out all this complexity in an organized way that hopefully illuminates dignity for what it is or for what it appears to be. This allows us to form a working foundation for studying it within American society.

## Relatively Speaking: Dignity Positioned against Proposed Synonyms

Recent years suggest a possible resurgence of "dignity" within public discourse. For instance, a Google N-gram analysis supports an upward tick in "dignity" in the past decade across tens of thousands of published texts.[1] Apparently, dignity's appeal exists across any partisan or ideological divides. In a joint session of Congress on April 28, 2021, President Biden asked, "Can our democracy deliver on its promise that all of us, created equal in the image of God, have a chance to lead lives of dignity, respect, and possibility?" Meanwhile, former president Donald Trump's farewell address claimed that "every citizen is entitled to equal dignity."

According to Merriam-Webster, dignity is "formal reserve or seriousness of manner, appearance, or language" or "the quality or state of being worthy, honored, or esteemed." However, dignity also refers to "high rank, office, or position." As the philosopher Remy Debes (2009) suggests at necessary length: "Dignity has also been pervasively conceived as honor, rank, station, inherent worth, inalienable worth, equal worth, supreme worth, uniqueness,

---

[1] A recent piece using N-gram statistics came to a similar conclusion, linking a rise in mentions of liberalism to a rise in mentions of human dignity (Nicole Yeatman, "A Brief History of Human Dignity," Big Think, November 30, 2020). The text corpus used for N-gram is not a direct indication of typical frequency of usage in everyday speech. Google trends, a site capturing all searches around the world, shows a similar pattern: searches since 2004 seem to have a slight upward trend with spikes around the times of notable world events like the Arab Spring and the US Black Lives Matter protests.

beauty, poise, gravitas, personality, integrity, bodily integrity, self-respect, self-esteem, a sacred place in the order of things." Across these wide-ranging definitions, we can start to appreciate some of the paradoxical aspects of dignity: dignity both is and is not about particular statuses held in society.

Is dignity an inefficient placeholder (e.g., Bagaric and Allan 2006): that is, a vacuous concept that should be replaced by clearer terms, depending on which specific aspects of "dignity" are at stake? Or a "useless" (Byk 2014) term? Relatedly, Pinker (2008) suggests (in an article titled "The Stupidity of Dignity") that dignity is "relative, fungible and often harmful: it's the sizzle, not the steak."[2] Pinker calls dignity a "squishy, subjective notion" that is appropriated by those on either side of power or legal divides to justify their causes. Yet, Pinker also says dignity deserves "a measure of cautious respect": without it, he says, one might "loosen his inhibitions against mistreating the [a] person." Even some of its critics, it seems, come around to respecting the term's rhetorical power across time and circumstance.

Within a recent edited volume, Malpas and Lickiss (2007) follow the tradition of illuminating dignity's dynamic embeddedness within "a network of concepts." Similarly, the British sociologist Andrew Sayer advocates an illumination of dignity in terms of how it is like or differs from other moral concepts, such as respect, status, charisma, or compassion. For instance, because dignity might be more understood than felt, it seems immediately different from sympathy (Hodgkiss 2018).

If we follow most politicians and social theorists, by assuming that dignity involves ongoing social relations and therefore is not always guaranteed or permanent, then what counts as dignified conduct will depend on the statuses or roles of the individuals involved. For example, presidents are expected to act differently from teachers, who in turn act differently from children; roles set expectations for the kind of conduct we are willing to accept, as the sociologist Erving Goffman so famously illustrated in *The Presentation of Self in Everyday Life*.

Notions of inequality and status were more central to older conceptions of dignity and are glossed over in many modern discussions. In fact, Debes (2017a, 2017b) suggests that our ancestors would be surprised by modern

---

[2] He continues: "What ultimately matters is respect for the person, not the perceptual signals that typically trigger it. Indeed, the gap between perception and reality makes us vulnerable to dignity illusions. We may be impressed by signs of dignity without underlying merit, as in the tin-pot dictator, and fail to recognize merit in a person who has been stripped of the signs of dignity, such as a pauper or refugee."

Western notions of dignity referring to some sort of universal human worth. Latin and French equivalents of dignity—*dignitas* and *dignités*—refer to a sense of social rank more than any sort of universal property of human life. "In other words, until a little over a century ago, dignity connoted social status of the kind associated with nobility, power, gentlemanly comportment, or preferment within the church—not some fundamental, unearned, equally shared moral status among humans" (1). In present-day, democratic societies, hierarchical or aristocratic notions of dignity that emphasize occupying one's proper place in society or behaving in a civil fashion might be closer to "honor" than "dignity," although status and inequality undeniably structure social relations even today (see Lindemann 2015).

What, then, sets dignity apart as a concept? Does it mean something different than its apparent synonyms? In the *British Medical Journal* in 2003, Dr. Ruth Macklin suggested that a notion of "dignity" needlessly—even "useless[ly]"—complicates medical ethics, because it means "no more" than "respect for persons or their autonomy." We can, she suggests, be good to our patients without getting bogged down in abstract debates. Seven years later, in the *Journal of Medical Ethics*, the philosopher Suzy Killmister called dignity "not such a useless concept," writing that dignity's "multiple strands" become unified by "understanding dignity as the capacity to live by one's standards and principles" (2010, 160).

Following Macklin and Killmister, is dignity just some minimal or essential form of autonomy? Autonomy, by itself, comes closer to sovereignty, or a power to be self-determining as an individual, group, or state (Resnik and Suk 2003). However, autonomy is a social project, not only in the sense of the social construction of persons as individuals who are unique, but also in the sense of the "nature of the autonomy that belongs to human being depend[ing] upon the nature of the human being that is autonomous" (Malpas 2007, 22). Similarly, consider how Nelson Mandela thought of freedom in relational terms: "For to be free is not merely to cast off one's chains, but to live in a way that respects and enhances the freedom of others."

More broadly, autonomy in a relational context of not respecting humanity might mean autonomy to further one's own ends while not supporting others'; it might even mean the freedom to discriminate, as the American Civil Liberties Union recently pointed out in drawing a connection between discrimination and "religious liberty," and as African Americans, Asian Americans, Native Americans, Latinx, and other individuals have identified as what it means to be marginalized in a "free country."

As the sociologist Robert Bellah and his colleagues suggested in 1985 in *Habits of the Heart*, a landmark study of American lives, "dignity only is achieved by becoming a respected member of a community knit together by mutual trust." Similarly, in a piece for the *Harvard Business Review*,[3] sociologist Andrew Sayer positioned dignity as achieved through "a mix of independence and interdependence," involving "recognition and trust, as well as autonomy and self-mastery." "In dignified work relations," for example, "people carefully avoid taking advantage of the inherent vulnerability of the employment relationship."

Aretha Franklin asked listeners to find out what respect means to her, and she defined it in terms asking a partner to "give me my propers when you get home." However, dignity is not just about social procedures of autonomy or respect, but also about a process of "being" (Lamont 2019) within a larger community that ultimately enriches and plays a role in defining one's self.

## Capturing Light in a Bottle: Is It Useful to Try to Pin Dignity Down?

Stepping back, why is there even an impulse to formally define what dignity means, rather than simply experiencing its changing or felt meanings across time, history, and individual lives? In part, the lexicographic impulse is necessary and understandable: for civilization to continue going on, we need to protect lives from violence and destruction. Dignity may well play a part in that, if there is enough consensus about what it means, and this can be formalized into norms, laws, or procedures.

Dictionaries only can do so much. Situational pressures often elude words or formal logic, instead belonging to the realm of embodied practice (e.g., Bourdieu 1990; Joas 1996; Lizardo 2017). What makes us feel guilt-stricken or proud or embarrassed or horrible or cool can be hard to put into words. However, to others who have experienced a similar situation, words or gestures might communicate roughly what we want to say, speaking to how experience grounds words and, by extension, how the discursive is interpreted in terms of the practical (Bourdieu 1990; Lakoff and Johnson 1999).

---

[3] Monique Valcour, "Managing People: The Power of Dignity in the Workplace," *Harvard Business Review*, 2014. https://hbr.org/2014/04/the-power-of-dignity-in-the-workplace.

Like light, dignity might only gain meaning or definition against context. For instance, a phrasal approach to dignity shows how it gains specific meanings through its intentional insertion next to other words, as in "dignity of body," "secular dignity," "losing one's dignity," "religious dignity," "dying with dignity," and so forth (Sayer 2007, 2011; Sennett 2003). "Carrying oneself with dignity" and "beneath one's dignity" point to the more status-oriented properties of the term; the former is associated with an "emotionally restrained"[4] or educated disposition, while the latter supposes a deserved treatment based on one's present status in life. In *Democracy in America,* Alexis de Tocqueville wrote that "true dignity in manners consists in always taking one's proper station, neither too high nor too low."

By insisting on definitional absolutes about dignity, researchers might unintentionally play into an unproductive tendency toward glib or superficial universalisms about irreducible, subjective experiences in historical and cultural context. To quote the sociologist John Levi Martin (2011), one gulf between academic theory and everyday experience takes the form of "the abstract answer that overrides the everyday knowledge of actors" (6). For example, is having a dignified appearance in a photograph the same thing as portraying dignity itself? Hardly. Bob Dylan wrote a song about how dignity has never been photographed. Similarly, an episode of *The Simpsons* involved a Pictionary skit where trying to draw "dignity" was a complete failure. Yet, with dignity, we still claim to "know it when we see it."

As we have learned from cultural sociology, what people say about what they think is not always a clear indicator of how they think in practical terms—that is, across different, applied contexts (e.g., Vaisey 2009; Rinaldo and Guhin 2019). All of this is to say that any hunt for a declarative or discursive definition of dignity devoid of context might be an intellectual or philosophical fantasy doomed from the start, based on the strong presumption that dignity would have any real substance apart from specific contexts. By analogy, the sociology of morality shifts the focus toward conceptions of morality within specific contexts of action or difficult contingencies individuals face, in place of universalistic or acontextual views on morality (Hitlin and Vaisey 2013; Luft 2020).

One learns about, and comes to define, ideas and ideals only through a generalization of concrete examples. As social psychologists, we believe that dignity fuses individuality and society through a route of moralized, practical

---

[4] Sennett and Cobb [1972] 1993.

creativity, which is a case we make in Chapter 3 when we talk about what it means to care for others beyond reason. Dignity may not be "real" in the neurological sense of pointing to it on a magnetic resonance imaging (MRI) scan, but people treat it as if it is a "real" ideal, something toward which we can strive in given moments, across lifetimes, and across the centuries.

Excepting human rights violations, there may be no ideal type of Dignity, but only dignities, or concrete realizations of dignity in given historical, cultural, and interpersonal contexts. Across these dignities, perhaps the only universal worth noting about dignity proper is that it always represents some accepted or desired relationship between self and society. This points to a fundamental paradox for dignity: it means different things to different people at different times, and yet still appears to cohere as a larger concept across time and space, even a tangible one. Dignity is bundled, somehow.

## Dignity as a Shifting Bundle of Moral Concepts: The Conceptual and Social Relationality of Dignity

Whether a concept is "real" and whether it can be formally defined are entirely separate issues. If dignity is experienced across time and people as a variable set of conceptions about individuals and their societies, then a specific definition may not be forthcoming, even as dignity remains important and real. To call a concept "vague" is not to rule out its real power, importance, or essentiality.

By "begging the question" of dignity, we might in fact begin to realize the pivotal, great nature of what we are asking about in the first place (Malpas and Lickiss 2007). That is, rather than undermining the importance or conceptual integrity of dignity, perhaps these definitional debates actually serve to highlight dignity's importance. Indeed, we are reminded of how other bedrock, powerful concepts, such as truth, goodness, life, or love, cause ferocious debate about definitions because of—not despite— their social importance. Like dignity, these concepts seem to be relational concepts, definable only *relative* to or within the midst of experience. Precisely *because* the concept is so important, people approach dignity in differing ways, mobilizing different elements or vocabularies relevant to dignity at differing times.

Like love, dignity is hard to define, and similarly is experienced and communicated as a bundle of moral concepts. In *Talk of Love,* the cultural sociologist Ann Swidler's (2001) respondents had plenty to say about "love," even if it was a series of contradictions and oft-inarticulate expressions of bafflement and wonder. Love's power resides not in a universality of definition, but in the multitude of definitions, and, perhaps even more, in the liberty of individuals to create their own individualized definitions or practices of love that resonate with those whom they love. Love is represented as a "toolkit" of meanings, images, metaphors, and vocabularies that mediate our experience of it as an abstract, timeless entity (see also Swidler 1986). Love means what it does to those who love and yet love is not so personal that we cannot talk about it meaningfully, as if it is universal in character. We talk about it and experience it as a singular concept existing beyond—transcending—its particularities.

## Intrinsic, Attributed, Inflorescent: Distinguishing Types of Dignity

Dignity, across its multiple manifestations, resides in a separation of who someone "is" from how they are treated and who they might become. Intrinsic dignity of belonging to humankind is apart from attributed dignity, which may or may not be denied or given socially. Intrinsic dignity rests in a human or species status; attributed dignity in social interaction or societal operations; and inflorescent dignity in potential that could lead to flourishing (e.g., Hodgkiss 2018; Sulmasy 2007). To paraphrase the professor of law and philosophy Jeremy Waldron (2009), dignity refers both to the status of human life and to the contingent, fragile realization of that same human status. Whereas intrinsic dignity is "a prerequisite of social interaction itself," attributed dignity is, in a performative sense, a "negotiated outcome of social interaction" (Callero 2014, 276). Intrinsically, dignity may function as that Simmelian widest circle of society: a social identity attached to the status of being human within a democratic society, or what Berger (1970, 342) called "humanity divested of all socially imposed roles or norms" and what Charles Taylor viewed as the experience of being a free, reasoning human subject who is creative and can work toward perceived moral goods or projects (Calhoun 1991). Metz (2014) argues that in many precolonial African societies, the notion of "ubuntu" represented a moral personhood through being part of society, a given and deep humanity, and a collective orientation less common in the modern West.

Similarly, when the philosopher Arthur Schopenhauer objected to dignity, he was objecting more to the sprawling if irreverent uses of the term, such as wide appropriations of the phrase "dignity of man," which he perhaps heard as armchair gestures toward morality. Crucially, he objected less to the existence of dignity itself. In fact, Schopenhauer seems quite amenable to confirming both the existence and importance of dignity in some *intrinsic* form: "immediately, and without reasons or arguments, that in-itself of his own phenomenon is also that of others," he writes. Thus, there is something in ourselves that exists for itself and that we also see when we look at others: many scholars would call this dignity. Because Schopenhauer also viewed this "in-itself" as orienting compassion and morality, something like dignity figured prominently in Schopenhauer's philosophy even if not labeled as such.[5]

Scholars are divided on whether dignity refers to the status of humans or the quintessence of life more broadly. For instance, referring to all animate matter, Aquinas refers to the dignity of a given life form in terms of its place within a larger, divine order (Rosen 2012, 17). In a conceptually similar way, Pico della Mirandola and Blaise Pascal grant humanity a distinctive existential status, though approach the matter somewhat differently. For Pascal, humanity's dignity is not in an idealistic moral rationality as it might be for della Mirandola, but rather comes from the capacity to know a larger context beyond one's potential misfortunes: in other words, to be capable of seeing beyond one's fate, perhaps not unlike how Sisyphus did in a way that enabled him to scorn his interminable megalithic task. In this way, one is always something—someone—more than one's present self.

Similarly, American medical ethicist Dr. Daniel Sulmasy (2007) calls dignity a "modest essentialism" that resists an idealistic essentialism in the sense of apartness from society, perception, or circumstance. According to Sulmasy and others, intrinsic dignity "inheres in the emergent constitution of personhood" and is "objective and ontologically real" (Smith 2009, quoted in Callero 2014, 276). In this vein, Sulmasy (2007) applies the philosophical concept of "natural kind" to "inherent dignity," drawing an analogy to bananas: green bananas and ripe bananas both are bananas and evoke a response as bananas. Thus, while subcategories indeed might complicate our

---

[5] Beyond philosophy, many major religions, including Catholicism, rest upon the inherent dignity of human life, such as through being a "child of God" or created in God's image. Baylor sociologist Laura Upenieks (2022) develops this idea in a recent paper on mental health when attachment to God falters.

response to kind, these subcategories would be fundamentally meaningless without any larger reference to kind—that is, without an overarching classification as "banana" or "human" in the first place (see also Monk 2022).

An attributed form of dignity differs from its intrinsic sense. This type of dignity rests within the constant flow of social interaction, as it captures the ongoing, perpetual sense of judgment humans have for one another. One can see the sharp contrast between what people want for themselves and what others want for them in moments of oppression or suffering, when dignity's purported intrinsic quality is denied or dismissed. Some people, to some people, are rendered outside of a circle of respect (Crimston et al., 2018). An interaction order (Goffman 1983), and social interaction in general, is based on the treatment owed to certain persons belonging to certain categories precisely on the bases of these categorical memberships but also, in many circles, simply by virtue of being human. When someone claims to be a certain kind of person, such as a person of a specific status or profession, we treat them in kind, or we can choose not to assent to their identity claim and risk offending them. One's dignity in life crucially depends, then, on others accepting their claims (Goffman 1959). We smooth over social interaction by extending what Goffman calls "tact" toward those who make small breaches.

Even while the sociologist of religion Christian Smith (2009) construes of dignity as a brute fact of personhood that remains amid physical incapacitation, the cultural sociologist Michèle Lamont and colleagues (2016) conceive of dignity as a continual coping process drawing on moral boundaries between ourselves and others. Similarly, the political philosopher Michael Rosen (2012, 14) offers the example of Cicero, who used dignity in at least two distinct senses: as acting according to one's social standing and as a way of understanding the species status of humans more generally within the realm of all earthly life.

In devaluing life, one makes the decision to strip it of its intrinsic value, as is often encountered during times of war or genocide when might overpowers humanity (Luft 2020, 2022). Christopher Columbus used Eurocentric conquest to justify possession of Native American land, lives, and culture. Thus, Columbus illustrates Sulmasy's stark contrast between intrinsic dignity and attributed dignity: Columbus saw intrinsic dignity—one cannot not see it[6]— and then chose to deny it.

---

[6] Even violence involves a recognition of others as human. After that human recognition, the importance of the recognition can be denied as justification for harm or murder.

Beyond this, there is inflorescent dignity—in the sense of "flowering" (Sulmasy 2013)—a sense of who we might become if given the social opportunity to excel or flourish. For instance, St. Thomas Aquinas spoke of "dignities" or favorable, promising attributes of individual lives, apart from Dignity itself (Düwell et al. 2014). We realize not only from within our own minds, as possible selves, but also by comparing or relating ourselves to others around us or who came before us what our potential might be. Limited cultures convey limited images of such potential. The crucial point, as Sulmasy argues, is that attributed and inflorescent dignities make no sense in the absence of intrinsic dignity, which is designated to us—to each of us— as part of humankind.

To simultaneously appreciate these senses of dignity, consider the intricacies involved in the seemingly simple realization that someone is ill. To realize that someone is not well, we must perceive that person as human, and then in terms of other people we know who we categorize as not sick. Thirdly, we also must understand how sickness stands in the way of realization of personal or human potential.

## In the Eye of the Beholder: Problems of Perspective Associated with Dignity

Discussions about dignity, academic or otherwise, depend not only on one's perspective or social location but also on prevailing assumptions about human nature, epistemology, and the nature of social organization. This renders the topic both difficult and central to understanding the nexus of people and society. To paraphrase diplomatic negotiations expert Donna Hicks (2011), dignity could denote a "birthright" to which each of us is socially entitled, its inherent form as just discussed. However, as Hicks notes, dignity also refers to a set of transactional, practical, hard-to-define procedures for making each other feel recognized and heard in ways that might become clear as a situation unfolds. In this regard, dignity's complex interactional properties render Hicks used to world leaders walking out of rooms in disdain even when the atmosphere is ostensibly "respectful" or "polite," suggesting that dignity might be something more than just gestures of "respect," itself a complicated set of behaviors and rituals that involve distinctions based on perceived status and experience. In asking what dignity "is," we inquire about generalities and specificities surrounding the concept, as well as differing conceptions of it. The term, despite its ineffability and even potential self-contradiction, endures.

One's own sense of right and wrong is not an academic question (Lukes 2008): it is experienced first-person as self-evidently true (see also Joas 2000). Waldron (2015, 92) writes: "Dignity, then, requires individuals to be allowed the power of choice over matters that they consider to be of the highest importance to themselves." Somewhat in contrast, Thomas Hobbes insisted in *Leviathan* that dignity is the "public worth of a man, which is the value set on him by the commonwealth," thus highlighting the third-person capacity to assign dignity to others regardless of what they think.[7] Similarly, Veblen observes in Wrong (1961, 190) that "the usual basis of self-respect is the respect accorded by one's neighbors." This points to a distinction between experience and analysis that will be important for our ongoing discussion: the same social phenomena can be experienced (and studied) from a first-person perspective or from the vantage points of third or outside parties. Reciprocally, a distinction between first- and third-person viewpoints creates a window for perceived discrimination and injustice to matter to dignity even if systems do not recognize such ills. Many Americans experience harms that can also be studied from the outside, a third-person understanding of first-person experiences that points to shared understandings of what matters and for whom.

Dignity can be a tool put toward social harm. Friedrich Nietzsche mocked the concept of dignity, a tool of demagogues blinding us to social elites, or even as a willful ignorance that might lead us to ignore the reality of deep existential suffering (Rosen 2012). Before the twentieth century, Karl Marx worried that an abstraction like dignity would steal attention away from the truly constraining material conditions of our difficult social existence. The Harvard psychologist Steven Pinker (2008) has pointed out how "dignity" has been used across the centuries as a Trojan Horse to further nationalist, inhumane, or eugenic agendas. Some uses of the dignity concept across the centuries and even today have rightly been called out when used to justify violence or hatred. Dignity, while sometimes used antisocially, has pointed eventual ways toward social or moral goodness.

Is there some inner, Archimedean capacity for salvaging dignity, even in the most horrific of circumstances? Wouldn't that also depend on

---

[7] Prior to modernity, Hobbes' postulation of dignity in terms of "public worth" set by a commonwealth is close to the Humean notion of "a noble dignity," in the case of the propertied classes (see Düwell et al. 2014).

whether one takes the individual's or an observer's point of view? Viktor Frankl, a Holocaust prisoner and renowned psychiatrist, began to envision a logotherapeutic approach while at Auschwitz-Birkenau, insisting that individuals can control how they construct meaning even when all of life's basic possibilities are threatened. Frankl stresses that having a "why" or reason to live weathers almost any "how" or trying circumstances necessary for survival. Scholars of marginalization have claimed that when one's life is not valued, or when one's suffering is actively promoted by society, self-preservation and even self-care take on more explicitly political dimensions, as a way of resisting larger forces of discrimination, hate, or genocide.

The dignity of an individual and their life can be at odds with what is deemed necessary to the dignity of a collective: war is employed as a ruthless tool for preserving sovereignty at the expense of individual lives. Groups and nations have asserted specific others as anathema to their moral codes or as threats to their very existence, thus placing individuals into situations where they kill or commit genocide for the purpose of self-preservation or group solidarity or often both (Luft 2020, 2022). However, "given the nesting of dignity in personhood, the Supreme Court's insistence on attributing dignity to states is seen by some as either obnoxious or disingenuous," in turn raising the vital question of to which levels of social and material reality dignity ought to pertain (Resnik and Suk 2003, 1926).

Judaism remembers the Holocaust in a way that uses collective memory as a device for collective dignity: by not forgetting names, we remember suffering and thus chart a better future. Lives lost are lives that existed and continue to exist through the radiating, living effects of their actions. Recent projects in the American South and in Canada have identified enslaved or Indigenous individuals whose bodies were left in mass graves. Through memory and vigil, communities can work toward dignifying deaths that occurred under the most undignified of circumstances, in the same way that societies can recognize and understand history and in doing so choose to redirect the future. Prisoners, the unhoused, and victims of autocracy can, through their continued, breathing existence, or through their composure, protest, or meaning making, demonstrate their dignity. Many who are called heroes or who lead social movements find themselves oppressed or taken as prisoners, and their dignity often seems to shine—rather than disappear—during these pivotal movements of resistance.

Whatever shape dignity takes depends on time: growth, resilience, and social change are trajectories—not snapshots. Dignity might rest in the moral actions of a life as they told to others, even as morality betrays life. To para-phrase Kierkegaard, narrating a story about one's life gives a person "eternal dignity" by translating social happenings into biographical events. Dignity in storytelling comes from how narration legitimates or consoles. Indignities inflicted cannot be undone, but some dignity can be restored if later words and actions proceed well, which is the subject of a field of international law focused on dignity restoration in South Africa (Atuahene 2016).

The notion of dignity has been invoked in social discussions of "dying with dignity" (Buchbinder 2021). This issue is experiencing a resurgence with increased implementation of assisted suicide or medical aid-in-dying. According to the sociologist and physician Nicholas Christakis' (2007) re-view of patient and provider survey data, what patients want for themselves during their final months of life is often different from what doctors think they want. Based on the available data, doctors often misestimate the amount of time patients have left when they are within their last year of life. What patients want is a function of the information that they are given about their remaining time left. Christakis recounts an episode in which *recognition* is what the patient wanted: the patient wanted to recognize their doctor as human by talking with them about their life and their family, and in that way to experience an undeniable human connection between two humans that, by its own essential dynamics, yields a sense of dignity.

Raphael's (1994) assertion that "dignity is required for being the object of a duty" allows for reframing animal rights in terms of the dignity of animals (as discussed in Hodgkiss 2018), raising the question of whether dignities can be compared or contrasted across life forms, as when ceremonial burial is given to a human but not to a pet. To consider the interaction of two dignities, consider how we might judge an individual after learning that he has pur-posely killed or eaten a dog or a cat. Thus, Hodgkiss (2018, 6) writes: "A loss of human dignity coming by way of mistreatment of our fellow non-human creatures has counterpointed the very idea of an exclusive human dignity." Through trans-species and within-species interaction, one is confronted with the essential property that dignity is based on interaction among lives *as much as* what one does or wills to do with one's own individual life, on one's own terms.

As Michael Rosen (2012) observes, there is in modernity a *noblesse oblige* when it comes to the dignified conduct of those in power. The powerful, given the influence with which they are vested, ought to be obligated to be kind to those of lesser status, whereas ordinary individuals should be entitled to disagreement or protest as a way of ensuring the stability of their relatively more economically and socially precarious existence. Centuries ago, the opposite trend prevailed by aristocracy, but the question remains as to whether voters will remain societal stakeholders throughout the twenty-first century.

Sisyphus manages to smile at his interminable and repetitive fate: by being able to think beyond it even if he cannot physically exist beyond it. A sense of perspective in the face of major or unchanging obstacles surely deserves closer attention as a basis of how individuals achieve dignity. Tocqueville called democracy "wanting": nowadays, the question arises as to how one upholds individual dignity when collective dignity is less forthcoming, such as in a milieu of inequality and polarization.

Even within the Ivory Tower, much of what dignity is literally is "lost in translation." For instance, Kantian understandings of dignity rest largely on the translation of German *würde* or "worth," which itself is a particular sense of dignity rather than dignity per se (Rosen 2012). A cross-cultural quest to find the "equivalent" of dignity or the "nearest approximation" of the term within a language or culture is bound to fail, not only due to anthropological problems of cross-cultural comparison resting on idiosyncratically valuable local meanings, but also due to the implicit centering of "normal" definitions within such scholarly quests. "Near-equivalents" to dignity, such as the French *dignités*, can have surprisingly narrow translations, in this case to "privileges" during the ancien régime.

## A Sociological Critique of Kantian Approaches to Dignity

There perhaps is no perspective on dignity more influential than Immanuel Kant's. Shared across the centuries and across countless, multidisciplinary writings on dignity, Kant's perspective places rationality and morality front and center in what dignity means and how it operates. In fact, Kant spoke of morality itself, not living a moral life per se, as the basis of human dignity. In the next few pages, we unpack Kant's perspective sociologically, not in terms of a formal philosophical analysis, but rather in terms of how Kant often is understood by many cultural, legal, and academic audiences. These prevailing understandings are likely to carry significant implications for how we research dignity.

Many credit Immanuel Kant with the philosophical shift toward basing intrinsic dignity on the potential for human autonomy through the exercise of reason or, more precisely, rational morality (Sensen 2011). This rational morality on doing only what one would mandate that others would do in one's situation is often termed "the categorical imperative" or Golden Rule of Kantian morality: "Act only in accordance with that maxim through which you can at the same time will that it become a universal law." Kant and his intellectual circle inhabit a life of the mind—of *philosophia*, or love of wisdom—and by recasting a purposeful life in terms of a rational life one might unfairly leave out many lives for which people are not "paid to think" (to quote Meryl Streep's forceful line from the recent film adaptation of *Little Women*).[8]

As far as a sociological perspective is concerned, a Kantian notion of only acting insofar as one would generalize one's actions for others to perform could be interpreted an implausible—and even dangerous—merger of egotism and universalism, precisely not the characteristics of dignity we find most plausible. Perhaps in a move toward pragmatism that we take in Chapter 3, we could attach this moral obligation to a shared definition of the situation, as doing the right thing might depend on what is at stake and for whom. The very "feel for the game" that renders a person an acceptable-to-others member of a social group relies on *not* abstracting from personal experience but, rather, demonstrating that you implicitly understand what your local group considers right, wrong, weird, or normal (Eliasoph and Lichterman 2003). If one is to always do what one would have anyone do in one's situation, then one would have little room for error, or a lot of room, depending on how seriously one takes the human mind's bottomless, brilliant capacity for self-justification and post hoc rationalization. Modern psychology, and classic sociological notions of self-serving "accounts," complicate this categorical imperative.[9]

Kant makes a separate point that "autonomy is therefore the ground of the dignity of human nature," seeming to suggest that autonomy and rationality are wedded through that magnificent apparent phenomenon of a "free-thinking human mind." Other than the phenomenological sense that one is the person who has one's thoughts, it is difficult to see how autonomy

---

[8] We often note in our graduate seminars the peculiar nature, relative to what most people in history have done most of the time, of those paid to ruminate about texts like this.

[9] As the comedian and amateur ethicist Michael Schur captures it, in addition to Kant's imperative process taking a long time and being a poor guide to necessary in-the-moment thinking, the fact that "behaving ethically can be a 'trust your gut' type of exercise, and Kant is here to tell us our guts are stupid and we shouldn't listen to them" (Schur 2022, 69–70), suggests Kant has little to say about how actual humans render actual moral judgment in actual situations.

and rationality are necessarily related. While autonomy has a potentially important role to play in dignity, most scholars of dignity emphasize its basis in social understandings of what makes somebody autonomous—different eras, places, and situations have different notions of autonomy. Thus, a sociological view conceives of dignity as impossible without social structures that manufacture visions of autonomy. Experiences and valuations of autonomy vary considerably across societies, peoples, and situations, all in ways that seem to uphold and support—even necessarily—individual as well as collective visions of dignity. Beyond an existential or personal freedom to act contrary to social constraints (e.g., Hitlin and Elder 2007), the autonomy to live up to one's social commitments exists in both "tighter" and "looser" cultures (Gelfand et al. 2011), and similarly across societies varying in their divisions of labor or network structures (Merton 1934).

Kant stipulates that rational morality is how humans become ends in themselves or dignified (Rosen 2012, 21). Confusingly, however, morality according to Kant carries dignity independently of its incarnation. This is tautological at best, for the simple reason that humans are the only beings capable of apprehending or understanding morality according to Kant, making it pragmatically impossible for morality to exist on a plane higher than human thought.[10]

To better see a sociological absurdity to Kant's idealistic position on dignity, one might point out its ruthless Cartesian dualism: Kant speaks as if morality itself had a brain with which to think about itself.[11] This supraindividual notion that morality is a substance with a self-reflective mind is, well, strange. Why would morality "care" whether humans chose it if it is already transcendent? There also is a basic contradiction inherent to Kant's writing on morality, of course: Kant himself can write about morality only because he himself has experienced it—or the possibility of it—personally. Thus, any philosophical stipulation of morality as an ideal ultimately is rooted in practice and experience. Rather than Platonic or ethereal, it is more like, as Kant says, "the moral law within me."

---

[10] This tautology is a critique of idealism or transcendentalism as well. This is, as they say, outside of our bailiwick.

[11] Proponents of natural law might well use evolutionary arguments to reveal humans' capacity for morality through genetic dispositions for cerebral or prefrontal development, but these dispositions carry no value or independent existence outside of their incarnation or realization through human life. The current state of evolutionary theory on this front bases the capacity for morality within brain systems that evolved within social communities to handle interactional dilemmas but still require social development to unfold (e.g., Buchanan and Powell 2018; O'Madagain and Tomasello 2022).

A related sense in which Kant's perspective on dignity might be read as idealistic or ableist stems from its general ignorance of corporeality and downplaying of what Schopenhauer, Smith, and others would refer to as sentiment or compassion. A fixation on rationality would seem to presume both the presence and the unquestionable power of a specific set of mental capacities. As Professor Stephen Post (2022), winner of the Alzheimer's Association Distinguished Service Award, contends in his recent book *Dignity for Deeply Forgetful People: How Caregivers Can Meet the Challenges of Alzheimer's Disease*, American culture is marked by "hypercognitive values" including an emphasis on linear rationality and an overvaluation of independence, to the real detriment of valuing "other intact human qualities from consciousness to creativity." In fact, Post contends that the term "dementia" limits what we see when we see a person living with Alzheimer's. By instead referring to "deeply forgetful people," we "place these individuals on a spectrum of forgetfulness within the community of human dignity."[12]

In Chapter 3, neuroscience shows how intuition, emotion, and rationality are inextricably intertwined. In short, even if one wants to base their philosophical evidence on whatever "pure reason" (standing outside cultural understandings of logic, causality, and such) might be, psychological science demonstrates how that reason is, for corporeal humans, anchored in bodily, emotional processes, themselves shaped by experience and culture. One cannot anchor one's understanding of human thought on thought itself; emotion is inextricable and the two are mutually constitutive. It's turtles all the way down, to paraphrase Daniel Dennett's philosophy of consciousness, not to mention the sheer immensity of gut-brain connections (Mayer 2011). The importance of perspective becomes even more pivotal once one considers neurodiversity, such as how individuals with Asperger's syndrome perceive and manage threats to their dignity, thus further highlighting links between diverse subjectivities and diverse dignities (Koskinen, Stevanovic, and Peräkylä 2021).

As Rosen (2012) points out, Kant elsewhere engages with the notion of the sublime, or that which inspires awe, and he appears to connect sublimity to dignity as well, suggesting that the irrationality of the sublime may be an additional basis for dignity. One might glean an overall impression from Kant's texts that he privileges rationality in terms of understanding dignity but does

---

[12] Thank you to Wade Rowatt for bringing this book to our attention. These quotes are from Stephen Post's book summary prepared for Duke University's Monthly Spirituality and Health Research Seminar.

not altogether dismiss other ways of knowing, though these might be viewed more in terms of what they are not than what they are: that is, irrational sensations having, in his view, limited purchase on human dignity.

Following this false dichotomy, one instilled by idealistic separation of mind and body, a long-term intellectual project for understanding dignity has been trying to "rejoin" rational and irrational senses of the term to arrive at some more realistic understanding of what dignity might mean. Rosen reinvigorates this intellectual project when he quotes Kant on the reverential capacity of the human mind toward "the starry heavens above me," suggesting that the socially learned desire to think rationalistically might be at emotion's whim after all.[13] Building on this position, the philosopher Sarah Clark Miller (2017) proposes a relational reconsideration of dignity, stating that "the capacity to care" might be "considered a distinguishing moral power—as rationality often is—in light of which humans have dignity." We move toward a more relational, pragmatic perspective on dignity in Chapter 3.

Kant and the classic sociologist Emile Durkheim agree regarding dignity in at least two aspects. First, they both take a dualistic and idealistic approach, by positioning mind as separate from body, and therefore morality as distinct from humanity. Second, following their dualistic approaches, they posit sacred, dignifying essences over which each individual is rendered a mere physical guardian. For Durkheim, the soul is to be guarded, and for Kant, it is the moral personhood within each of us that needs to be protected. Durkheim, however, studies shared experiences of transcendence and meaning in a way that, we suggest, helps merge the social and the intuitive. We revisit some of Durkheim's scholarship in Chapter 2, as we build out our population health perspective on dignity.

### Individuals as Sacred: How Legal Frameworks Place Individual Lives in the Balance

Once determined by aristocratic hierarchies (Berger 1970; Rosen 2012; Taylor 1994),[14] dignity has also since become shorthand for the "status of

---

[13] We are swayed, incidentally, by the observation by Hans Joas (personal communication) that rationality is a "cultivated" form of human cognition that we can arrive at with practice and effort, but far from the default one and actually rather rare.

[14] *Dignitas* refers to Roman conceptions of (masculine) rank.

democratic citizenship" (Habermas 2010) or socially mediated autonomy (Hodgkiss 2013; Hodson 1996). As Habermas (2010) observed, dignity implies that individuals are, and ought to be treated as, ends, not as means toward ends, a core Kantian precept. Given this, dignity serves as a basis of moral codes, as Misztal (2013), Waldron (2009), Berger (1970), and others have observed in denoting dignity "a generalization of particularistic respect connected with rank and nobility" (Misztal 2013, 112).

The sociologist Philip Hodgkiss has noted, within many Western nations affected by global capitalism, a shift from *hierarchical* conceptions to *humanitarian* conceptions, what the sociologist of religion Peter Berger has labeled as "the obsolescence of honor" in favor of "identity and its intrinsic dignity apart from, and often against the institutional roles through which the individual expresses himself in society" (Berger 1970, 345). Habermas (2010) makes a similar point, writing on today's constitutional, legal democracies: "The concept of human dignity transfers the content of a morality of equal respect for everyone to the status order of citizens who derive their self-respect from the fact that they are recognized by all other citizens as subjects of equal actionable rights" (472). This is relatively new in human history; Debes (2017b) traces this back to between 1830 and 1850 and shifts from its English and Latin roots, a period that Joas (2011) agrees represents a positive shift in human understanding about the sacredness of the person. Our modern understanding is itself a social institution (Lindemann 2015).

Indeed, dignity is a "portal" through which modern conceptions of morality and individualism are "imported" into law (Habermas 2010). When we are confronted with the great fragmentation or differentiation of the various activities marking contemporary life, any notion of a collective good can easily be obscured.[15] More specifically, Luhmann (1965) links dignity to how individuals in modern societies take on multiple, diverse roles, thus necessitating an underlying personhood motivating and existing apart from particular roles (Neuhäuser and Sotecker 2014). Similarly, the sociologist Max Weber has argued that dignity shifts in Modernity toward a "dignity of personality."

Rosen (2012) and McCrudden (2013) both refer to an ethical decision-making example drawn from German law. In this example, the German constitution's emphasis on the dignity of the individual is referenced to reject the shooting down of a hijacked aircraft headed toward a civilian target.

---

[15] As Margaret Thatcher surmised, there is "no such thing as society."

Because individuals cannot be used as means, only ends, they cannot be gunned down for public safety, because they have not consented to the taking of their own lives.

While this example reminds us of the Trolley Dilemma in moral philosophy,[16] in which life is lost regardless of how one acts, the point here regarding dignity is that such calculations do not compute in terms of numbers even if we think they might: it is more like subtracting infinities from infinities even as we offer utilitarian summaries of numbers of lives saved. Because life is, by Kant, "beyond price," no computations with lives in the balance are ethically valid. Pragmatically, this point might seem hopelessly out of touch in today's world, too far removed from reality to be useful: lives have been, and always will be, on the line within tragic situations, and bystanders can intervene in ways that reduce loss of life even if some loss of life still occurs.

However, Rosen develops this example more usefully with the further reflection that a difference between shooting down and not shooting down a hijacked plane headed toward a civilian target is passengers who live an hour or two longer in abject terror, as death results to all on board in either scenario. When asked, would passengers on board consent to an earlier death in order to save hundreds or thousands of lives on the ground? Many likely would, thus showing how the enumeration of lives can still matter to dignity.

Of course, the plane example rests on certain or confident knowledge that the plane is headed toward a target and cannot be diverted, and it also assumes that control of the plane cannot be regained. These are observer suppositions made using tactical intelligence, and the stakes of the example completely change as these suppositions become more relaxed. For instance, if the plane could be taken back, no lives might be lost at all, either aboard or on the ground. Suppositions come from practical intelligence gained across past situations judged to be similar or highly similar, and all practical intelligence involves some degree of extrapolation. However, rejection of intelligence leads to negligence of duty, creating major problems.

As Rosen points out, a milder example would be from ordinary civilian life in societies with large numbers of guns, where an officer forcefully pushes down or restrains a civilian to keep them out of the line of active fire. This hardly seems like a moral dilemma. This would represent a momentary violation of physical dignity in the service of protecting a life. Many individuals

---

[16] "It's like the philosophy version of 'Stairway to Heaven' . . . an admitted classic that has suffered from overexposure" (Schur 2022, 40).

would likely be thankful for this in retrospect, raising the ethical question of how absence of willful consent might be "justified" or legitimated later, after the event, in a way that restores an overall sense of dignity to all parties involved. Not coincidentally, as Rosen points out, informed consent as a social institution has diffused widely across legal, scientific, and business contexts as a basic or minimal way of safeguarding the dignity of participants, subjects, or those with less power in given situations.

Transnational military strategy recognizes that some lives may be lost regardless of course—and the quantity of human loss therefore is to be *managed*. One might even extend a quantity-of-loss logic to the management of the Covid pandemic, as governments around the world recognized quite early on that a no-death scenario would be almost impossible and that infrastructure and resources should be marshaled in such a way that minimizes the loss of human life. Judging by Covid-19 mortality and infection rates, the pandemic added insult to pre-existing economic and health injuries within frontline workforces and marginalized communities and families (e.g., Anderson and Ray-Warren 2022; Janke et al. 2021; Verdery et al. 2020; Weinberger et al. 2020).

## Existing Sociological Research on Dignity: Definition Unknown

While disciplines such as philosophy, law, medicine, and public health have discussed dignity at considerable, impressive depth, it is rarer to investigate a dignity concept scientifically, with an eye toward measurement and replication. To be clear, many efforts in law or medicine use empirical, vital examples to anchor their particular conceptions of dignity (e.g., Jacobson 2007, 2012; Weinrib 2016). However, it is rare to revise and build theory on dignity based on broader processes of social interaction not involving basic, constitutional rights or major illness.

Sociology has made considerable progress in applying and developing the dignity concept in a broader set of practical, applied settings. Dignity is found in human relations that can be studied by social researchers. Relations are embedded within structures and networks of unequal power, status, resources, and opportunities. Sociologists such as Martha Crowley, Emile Durkheim, Erving Goffman, Randy Hodson, Michèle Lamont, Karl Marx,

Andrew Sayer, Richard Sennett, and Max Weber have made use of the dignity concept. These scholars often seem to suggest that dignity thrives on "tension" and "complementarity" between individuals and their work or labor contexts (Sayer 2007, 567), which echoes a broader sociological and even philosophical quest to understand how social order arises from individuals.

Arthur Schopenhauer thought dignity had become too widely used to mean anything concrete or valuable (Hodgkiss 2018). In this way, the multifariousness of dignity might have a useful or damning parallel in America's competing value structure. *However, as we argue in this book, differing conceptions of dignity are typical, and regardless they lead individuals to think carefully about what matters to them.*

Referring to a "cult of personal dignity," Durkheim (1972) suggests that it could exist to the detriment of other versions of faith: "It is still from society that it takes all its force, but it is not to society that it attaches us. . . . Hence, it does not constitute a true social bond" (146). Sanctimony toward individual lives, proffered by society itself, either overshadows or helps realize a God-given version of individual dignity. Meanwhile, Weberian notions of dignity focus on a fading subjective awareness in an era of rationalization and bureaucratization. Forces of nature or God are overshadowed by an incessant focus on productivity, racing toward presumed technological mastery of the environment. Our connections are with our local niches in organizations, less with society as a whole. However, religion's staying power in modern times is but one indicator that disenchantment is far from inevitable or absolute.

Lamont and colleagues (2016) suggest that dignity can be violated or reduced by discrimination, stigma, and other forms of social exclusion. However, they note, dignity also reflects the continual, motivated efforts of individuals to engage in boundary work: that is, reinterpret their circumstances and embed themselves in local networks and relationships that give their life value and purpose. By recasting higher-status social groups as having inhumane qualities or deciding they are less moral, oppressed, or lower-status individuals can reclaim themselves as humane, authentic, and thriving despite marginalization (see also Anderson and Snow 2001; Lamont 2000; Silva 2013). In short, the buffering of threatened dignity can depend on subcultures forged within wider social orders that are abrasive to the dignity of marginalized groups (e.g., Lamont 2000; Oeur 2016; Scott 1976; Wilcoxson and Moore 2020).

Ethnographic work on worker dignity (Lamont 2000) and interactional strategies among unhoused individuals (Anderson and Snow 1987) reveals ways that individuals distance themselves from others who marginalize or discredit them while embracing their own values in the process. Oeur (2016) recently showed how multiple dignities might involve a desire to be known in some situations and remain anonymous in others.

The move toward empirical investigation of dignity exists within recent, ethnographic research, a body of work that offers valuable insight in uncovering what fundamentally matters to a life well lived across distinct structural locations in society (e.g., Crowley 2013; Hodson 2001; Lamont 2000; Silva 2013). These studies focus on specific potential determinants of dignity, such as occupational conditions or racial, ethnic, or cultural boundaries (Crowley 2013, 2014; Hodgkiss 2015; Lamont et al. 2016).

While U.S. labor laws now prevent some forms of worker abuse, a range of work-related threats to dignity have attracted research attention. A related series of qualitative-comparative studies rooted in Lamont's (2000) *Dignity of Working Men* and Hodson's (2001) *Dignity at Work* revealed conditions that may uphold or undermine worker dignity. Drawing on over two hundred ethnographies, Hodson and Roscigno (2004) found that well-run organizations with employee involvement and a relative absence of employee abuse or disciplinary firings fared well on "worker dignity," measured as meaningful work and positive coworker relations. However, organizations that fared consistently poorly on these elements tended to undermine worker dignity, as did some organizations with contradictory combinations of elements.

Crowley (2013, 2014) conducted similar meta-analyses of worker ethnographies, examining worker dignity in terms of autonomy, creativity, and meaningfulness of work, as well as satisfaction, commitment, and effort at work. In terms of an erosion of dignity, Crowley focused on shame and co-worker conflict. As in Hodson and Roscigno's study, Crowley analyzed qualitative evidence from a wide swath of industries, occupations, and firms, spanning the diversity of the labor force. Crowley isolated the especially detrimental role of favoritism for generating coworker conflict and found on average that male work groups are afforded more rewarding work, while female work groups are more likely to experience coercion (such as direct supervision).

At a basic level, these studies document how—even though jobs and firms look profoundly different across professional, manual, and service occupations—certain principles either undermine or uphold employee dignity. An absence of abusive or coercive relations and ample, meaningful involvement of employees and availability of on-the-job training contributes to greater senses of worker dignity. Crowley (2013) also found that conditions of perceived dehumanization were more common in lower-status occupations. Thus, even though worker dignity might be based on some universal properties, it may be harder to experience at lower levels of socioeconomic status. There are specific behavioral avenues by which workers may glean dignity even when work conditions are coercive or demeaning, such as through withholding or rationing effort, bonding, organizing, or protesting (Hodson 1996; Crowley 2013).

This research is extremely useful for establishing multiple ways in which work conditions could relate to dignity. However, among those who study dignity at work, there is no clear consensus on what "dignity" per se means or to whom, or on how it might vary in how it is perceived. To define dignity in the context of work, Lamont (2000) cites Hodson (1996): "having autonomy for defining one's identity and protecting oneself from abuse." Roscigno, Yavorsky, and Quadlin (2021, 567) state: "Consensus, in fact, has begun to emerge that dignity is a multidimensional construct . . . and one that fundamentally rests on respect and recognition."

Following Roscigno and colleagues' recent analysis of U.S. General Social Survey data, there is much reason to think that outcomes such as respect at work, fairness in pay, fairness in promotions, and job satisfaction would both shape and reflect overall, subjective perceptions of dignity. We investigate empirical possibilities such as these in the second half of this book. Sharon Bolton has interviewed workers who claim that dignity, in addition to reflecting fairness and freedom from abuse, also relates to "little things," "pay," respect, or protection from unexpected demotion at work. But what resemblance does all this bear, exactly, to the widely cited Kantian or Cartesian emphases on staying "true to the moral sources which we find within us, and which are reached by the use of our reason" (Calhoun 1991, 255)? These wider, philosophical definitions—for their part—seem to suggest that particularities of how individuals realize what they want and relate to others in the process could be just as important to dignity. Also, while dignity at work is likely a core source of self-definition, at least for those who work or who have worked, it is but one domain in which people seek meaningful lives and a sense of social worth.

## What Do We Hope to Add to a Science of Dignity?

On the whole, recent research investigating the concept of dignity, mainly among workers, makes progress in uncovering different forms of interpersonal relations and how they matter. However, these studies do not empirically analyze dignity itself, often focusing on its specific determinants such as work or occupational conditions or racial or ethnic categories. These approaches make it difficult to develop cumulative scientific knowledge about the essence of dignity: how it is perceived socially, or how it is socially patterned.

If, as Lamont suggests, dignity reflects both structural oppression and boundary work pushing back against it, then what actual levels of dignity do we see in the world? How effective is boundary work against perceived indignity? More provocatively, following Marx, to what extent might workers internalize oppression as dignity, through situational forms of false consciousness that provide cognitive distraction from confronting objective obstacles within capitalism?

To paraphrase bell hooks, we aim in the coming chapters for something like a decolonization of the mind through making structural insidiousness more explicit: that is, by articulating multifaceted oppressions that might affect dignity or whether it is perceived as such. Multiple senses of dignity in America shape how individuals conduct themselves and think about their behavior as they relate to social, political, or legal ideals. These processes come to bear in how we might think about perceived levels of dignity. Ernest Hemingway once wrote, "You are so brave and quiet I forget you are suffering." Jesse Jackson observed quiet dignity in Jackie Robinson, who could not "punch back." While there is indignity in social devaluation, there could be some measure of dignity in social endurance, which we develop in the next chapter by recasting dignity as a form of social endurance reflecting both status and its lack.

We are witnessing a clear movement—within Western academic, legal, and political discourses—from status-oriented to individual-oriented social constructions of dignity, toward greater emphasis on the ways social systems can both enable and impinge on individuality. Despite the obvious benefits of this shift for individual safety, autonomy, and growth, it carries a social harm: to the extent that dignity is viewed in a "structure-free" way, electively or passively blind to obstacles most individuals face for social respect or economic mobility, it might be compared to a "color-blind" or antiseptic, philosophical stance on dignity, like Kant's. Structure-free views on dignity falsely imagine obstacles to be similar regardless of race, class, gender, age, or any other social structures. People's reports of their dignity, we argue, indicate facets of wider structures while also superseding them in the name of defining—and dignifying—individual lives.

# 2

# Seeing Circles

## Dignity as a Public Health Issue

As Andrew Sayer observed, dignity is "clearly important to people" despite its complicated nature. In this chapter, we defend dignity as worthy of scientific study. Following the last chapter, dignity involves social visions that societies, communities, and people construct given their moral commitments. Across these diverse dignities, a resounding theme is a calling-to-attention of how individuals and societies ought to relate in ways that uphold a vision of public health.

Borrowing from Georg Simmel, who distinguished social forms from their particular realizations, we can talk about the geometric properties of a circle apart from any specific circle. Similarly, instances of dignity call out experienced links between specific selves and various social circles that we can discuss separately from the broader idea of dignity as membership in the circle of humanity as a whole.

As we discuss here, each of these circles makes a difference to public health, ranging from close social ties to social categorizations to institutions and entire societies. Our focus on social ties and personal networks is developed more at length in Chapter 3, while links between categorizations and institutions receive greater focus in Chapter 4. Altogether, it is worth discussing arrangements of selves and social circles broadly, before getting into the specifics.

## The Sociological Imagination: Understanding Dignity at the Interface of Self and Society

Even with extensive, transhistorical variation in its details, a core of dignity remains constant. Dignity is about how societies and the individuals within them do or do not recognize and treat each other as legitimately human, based on local or social understandings of proper or sanctioned conduct.

*The Science of Dignity*. Steven Hitlin and Matthew A. Andersson, Oxford University Press.
© Oxford University Press 2023. DOI: 10.1093/oso/9780197743867.003.0003

Dignity, in short, is evident as a continual process of reimagining how societies and individuals ought to interface—a back-and-forth reconciling of societal structures with the needs, desires, and capabilities of those who live within these interwoven moral, social orders (Goffman 1983).

Dignity becomes a locus for getting a theoretical—and eventually empirical—handle on the problem of social order, as people strive to meet social standards. That is, dignity denotes a locally recognized humanity, one marked by autonomy, nonhumiliation, and the realization of locally defined social purpose (Habermas 2010; Hodson 2001; Lamont 2000; Misztal 2013). Social problems are social because they affect persons and vice versa, and dignity therefore captures the dialectical nature of how individuality is constructed and problematized in modern society.

Dignity, as experienced by people, incorporates situated morality as well as a judgment of one's life situation and direction. It used to be more based in rigid status differences. Even today, status remains a key aspect of dignity, in terms of who gets to define dignity and who notices, cares about, or remedies the absence of dignity. Moreover, social violence can be interpreted differently by individuals—or sometimes even not noticed if they become habituated to mistreatments within dehumanizing cultures. Yet, status and rank only tell part of the story of how dignity arises within a modern context.

## Suicide as a Lens for Understanding Individuals and Their Relations to Societies

If dignity is about how societies and individuals connect, then we might begin with the most extreme example of individuals disintegrating from society.[1] According to the World Health Organization, 1 in 100 deaths are by suicide.[2] Relatedly, a foundational study in sociology is *Suicide*, by Émile Durkheim. By reframing a personal, private decision as a socially patterned process, Durkheim posed a sociological investigation of whether to define suicide purely as "intentional self-homicide" (Porpora 2015) or as an indicator of patterns in wider social relationships. Durkheim relied on official suicide statistics to discover profound rate differences across demographic

---

[1] For one review, see Mueller et al. 2021.
[2] "One in 100 Deaths Is by Suicide," News Release, World Health Organization, June 17, 2021, https://www.who.int/news/item/17-06-2021-one-in-100-deaths-is-by-suicide.

groups and across countries. At the time he wrote, Protestants committed suicide more frequently than Catholics and the French more than the English.
The fact that suicide rates differ so profoundly across social groups organized
by class, gender, race, age, nationality, religion, and other characteristics has
provided evidence that suicide indeed is socially patterned; evidence of suicide clusters within social networks also points to the role of social influence
in these profoundly personal decisions (Mueller et al. 2021).

Durkheim positioned suicide as a loss of the dignity of an individual life.
That is, because each life is a human being, a being at once instilled and
recognized by society, killing the self is a murder of society. "Our dignity as
moral beings is therefore no longer the property of the city-state," Durkheim
wrote, "but it has not for that reason become our property, and we have not
acquired the right to do what we wish with it."[3]

Immanuel Kant apparently came to a similar conclusion, at least in terms
of his categorical imperative to do only what we might will others to do in
our same situation. Moreover, Kant saw personhood as the means by which
societies and individuals intersect: "The self-regarding duties are the supreme
condition and *principium* of all morality," he writes, "for the worth of the
person constitutes moral worth." For Kant, one loses dignity by "dishonoring
the humanity in one's person." As we will show later in this book, individuals
with lower levels of dignity also report some of the lowest levels of mental and
physical health, suggesting that deterioration of the self's vitality coincides
with deterioration of the self-society relationship that creates and gives legitimacy to the self in the first place.[4]

## Dignity Is Determined by Tensions between Societal, Group, and Individual Progress

Durkheim was one of the first sociologists to research population health. His
work underscores how individuals are based in webs of social relationships
and how individuals within some groups or populations are more vulnerable

---

[3] As quoted by Hecht 2013, 197.
[4] Fundamental questions of how much autonomy people have, versus social pressures, goes back a
long time (e.g., Wrong 1961) in sociology, with our peculiar (to Americans) hunch about the power
of the things outside of us that somehow shape us (e.g., Martin 2001). Many pages have been written
on the relative importance and/or intertwined nature of these poles of "structure" and "agency," some
by us, but the issues seem anecdotally to be fading now in light of larger societal inequities coming
even more prominently to the fore of the field.

based on both the nature and disintegration of these webs. Taking a similar viewpoint, epidemiologist and physician Sandro Galea recently suggested in a blog post that advancing health "starts with acknowledging both the harms that have been inflicted upon some populations and a celebration of all that we have in common."[5] "The starting place is respect and acceptance," he wrote, which sounds an awful lot like Durkheimian sacredness of individual and group life, and like putting dignity front and center in an approach to population health.

Even as average population health has improved remarkably across the preceding decades (Farmer et al. 2013), inequalities in health have remained and grown across and within populations (Link and Phelan 1995). Rising tides do not lift all boats. The enmeshment of average progress and growing inequality is central to fundamental cause theory, one of the central theories of health inequality in the epidemiological and social sciences (Link and Phelan 1995). This theory states that as health technology improves, so does population health. At the same time, however, well-resourced individuals have time, money, networks, and knowledge and are best poised to effectively utilize life-promoting technologies such as screenings, procedures, and pharmaceuticals. Hence, social progress and social inequality go hand in hand, with a small handful of exceptions involving great ease of access and low patient cost (Chang and Lauderdale 2009). More important, health inequalities are much more about what happens outside the walls of health care facilities, before individuals become patients, and here again well-resourced, higher-status individuals carry the advantage of residing in geographic areas with safer and greater work opportunities, neighborhoods, schools, community networks, and air and water quality (e.g., Heckman and Krueger 2003; Jackson 2015; Link and Phelan 1995; Mirowsky and Ross 2007; Williams and Mohammed 2013; Wilson 2012).

Deep tensions among social progress, group progress, and individual progress are fundamental to understanding dignity and health. For instance, as Durkheim originally envisioned, periods of rapid economic or social change can induce not only social inequality or unrest but also a broad sense of disorientation that makes individuals feel disconnected from social life.

How might we unite societal progress with the progress of groups and individuals within societies? In *Disrupting Dignity: Rethinking Power and*

---

[5] "How Love and Hate Influence Health and Racial Equity," *Culture of Health* (blog), Robert Wood Johnson Foundation, October 27, 2021.

*Progress within LGBTQ Lives*, Stephen Engel and Timothy Lyle (2021) offer one answer: we need to change the relationship between public health and marginalized groups. Marginalized and queer populations have too long endured being the subject of observation or research—or "public health interventions"—only to see their situations in society remain stigmatized or even worsened through harm or social exclusion. If science is going to help with population health, it needs to help with destigmatization along the way, as Matthew Clair, Caitlin Daniel, and Michèle Lamont (2016) have already observed. Hierarchy undercuts solidarity through differences in power and stigma. Webs of relationships become clustered in ways that undermine social coordination.

In *Dignity and Health*, Nora Jacobson (2012) poses solutions for reforming health care and social services based on an understanding of what dignity means to individuals. Courtesy and respect are concrete strategies for promoting dignity, according to interviews. A recognition of the importance of dignity is a needed starting point for reforming current standardized procedures and practices of clinical and social care that are based in narrow, rationalistic notions of patient time and resources (e.g., shuster 2016, 2022; Timmermans and Berg 2010). Patient-centered care has diffused throughout medical institutions, and the patient that it is designed to serve clinically often is divorced from the social contexts and socially caused illnesses it aims to heal (e.g., Freese and Lutfey 2011; Reynolds 2021).

Historically, scholars of dignity rightly have asked whether societies that condone prejudice, mass killings, poverty, or systematic genocide operate in ignorance of human dignity. The fact that societies exist and are stable at all—often remarkably stable, in fact—demonstrates what sociologists refer to as social order and social structure. Social structure is itself indisputable evidence for a social recognition—albeit still fundamentally flawed and categorically unequal—of each individual or a kind of human dignity. Social recognition rewrites and constructs hierarchies out of sheer, interpersonal recognition of humanness.

When Barack Obama and Neil deGrasse Tyson each quote Martin Luther King Jr. to liken contemporary society's changes to "an arc bending slowly toward justice," they are invoking a narrative of historical progress. Narratives of social progress tend to foreground an "average" or "typical" human experience, as discussed by the sociologists Louise Seamster and Victor Ray (2018). The progress-sayers are of course right in some ways, and they include prolific and well-known scholars inside and outside of academia, such as Steven

Pinker (2018), Hans Rosling (2018), and Paul Farmer and colleagues (2013), who in widely sold books have highlighted remarkable aggregate global progress in health, education, and financial well-being in the past century. Global poverty and infectious disease continue to decline, war is declining in frequency and severity, and globalization is bringing opportunity and democracy even as it elicits major challenges to the very humanity it supports. Diffusion of wealth through educational systems and labor markets spreads power and influence. People live longer and healthier lives and fewer people die in childbirth. Living in better health and with skills to offer to society are important inputs to human dignity. In short, some of Earth's so-called vital signs—excepting well-known countertrends such as atmospheric carbon dioxide, the strong grip of colonialism, and the runaway financialization of the world's economic elite—are trending favorably for many people.

Of course, structures of social dominance determine which groups shape prevalent narratives and understandings of history, self, and life. As we would expect, potentially favorable trends across society as a whole mask massive individual or group-based variation in resources, identity, and the attainment of justice. We engage these narratives as we draw links between societal structures and individual dignity.

Indeed, *which* vital signs to emphasize is a perhaps more important issue and one closer to the heart of dignity. As global capitalism predominates, how do we explain that peculiar moral phenomenon of thinking people deserve a better standard of living while also feeling structurally powerless to make it so? How do we explain the related, perhaps even more perplexing phenomena of feeling guilty for wanting to change a system that "already works" or of blaming ourselves for the suffering of our distant neighbors? We live in an era of mass incarceration and persistent inequality, one in which experiences and perceptions of discrimination correlate with depression, heart disease, and death, making the health consequences of inequality quite grave.

On the NPR podcast *Throughline*, an economist stated that "we all live like Louis XIV if not better," referring to the fact that the average standard of living has elevated considerably since the ancien régime. Shortly after, an emergency room nurse called into the show, which took place during the Covid pandemic, stating, "I'm trying not to kill my partner by sleeping in a different room, I work ungodly and unpredictable hours."[6] Clearly, averages and individual experiences tell completely different stories.

[6] "Capitalism: What Is It?," *Throughline*, National Public Radio, June 24, 2021, https://www.npr.org/transcripts/1008906741.

Dignity is based on cultural notions of how we should be living even if by some measures we live well.

Instead of population-wide averages standing in for a presumed human experience, we might instead imagine group-based fates, as is becoming increasingly common in population health and social sciences. That is, we shift from focusing on how society treats an "average" person—a conglomerate statistic representing no actual, real person—to an approach focused more on variation or sheer range in human experience, whether across social or demographic groups or variously situated individual persons.[7] Some might even inquire about the power relations inherent in who gets to decide "we," itself.

Viewed through the lens of inequities, a quest for human dignity operates more along the lines of what the trans poet Joshua Sassoon Orol (2019) stated: "No one is possible until everyone is. On this one truth, never compromise." If society is measured in terms of "average" experiences, one arrives at one set of conclusions; if society is measured in terms of its most marginalized or most elite,[8] conclusions are quite different in both scope and tenor. #AllLivesMatter imagines a kind of structure- and color-blind pseudoequity. That is, so the Panglossian story goes, all individuals already count, and are equally safe. By extension, individuals nowadays are not neglected by society, not in a post-civil rights era, not in one marked by quantum medical, technological, social, and legal advances relative to centuries before.

We need only look to Uvalde, Texas, in May 2022 to know that killings still make the news and shift policy discussions, even while the average person will not be murdered. Inequities of human experiences, rather than "average" experiences, are used to understand the state of society. Thus, average- and variation-oriented approaches to society are not contradictory but complementary: we use individuals to understand society as a whole. Dignity points to how averages and inequalities are part of the same picture, perhaps especially within democratic societies. The population health argument that we will be making in this book focuses on individuals' differing positions within capitalism and how those reflect historical differences in social and moral

---

[7] Inequities can be usefully distinguished from inequalities through a focus on social justice. Inequalities simply are mathematical deviations around a mean.

[8] The extremes matter: Nietzsche notably thought societies should be judged by the two or three greatest people they produced; if it took slavery and infanticide to get a Socrates and Aristotle, it was worthwhile.

Economic   →   Social
Inequality   ←   Inequality

**Figure 2.1** The Self-Reinforcing Relationship between Economic and Social Inequality

worth. Health unfolds across this entire process, in terms of the individual resources and stresses (Figure 2.1).

## Never Hierarchy-Free: The Perpetuation of Social Inequities through Status Characteristics

Belief systems change. Recently, privilege has been understood by many as a relative freedom from social oppression, such as not having one's access to social rights, institutions, or well-being rest upon specific Supreme Court decisions or the voting results of a particular state electorate. The longer one's social categories have remained free from restriction, the longer "people like you"[9] have had time—decades or centuries—to accumulate prestige, power, and wealth in America or elsewhere in the world.

As human rights scholars point out, modern notions of dignity compose a system anchored in fair treatment owed to individuals due to their intrinsic humanity. Vitally, this suggests that when we see someone, we see that they belong to a group in which all humans belong, and we should treat them accordingly. Individuals have an essence transcending their categories.

Yet, in practice, lives are treated unequally, and this too can be traced to how societies operate. When Simmel said we see each other as if through a veil, he meant that we never see the whole person. Situation by situation, we relate to other people by processing them categorically. Paradoxically, we parse entire individuals by parsing specific things about them (e.g., Stets and Burke 2000; Lamont et al. 2016; Levy et al. 2009; Ridgeway and Correll 2004).

No known civilization has existed hierarchy-free. Some form of hierarchy is part and parcel of social order. Living has always been a matter of navigating how one is valued in others' eyes, for better or worse. Audre Lorde observed that differences in themselves do not divide. It is society that divides, and it divides through the creation and perpetuation of hierarchy,

---

[9] "People like you" is a common phrasing in social surveys capturing a sense of group identity.

which, to continue applying Lorde's quote, creates "an inability to recognize, accept, and celebrate those differences."

Hierarchy assigns value to difference. Differences are differences when they carry social meaning as such. Lamont and other sociologists imagine heterarchy in its stead: a plurality of hierarchies, so that hierarchies of power and influence no longer are hegemonic, and each individual might glean substantive worth and value. Alternatively, in task-focused settings such as workplaces, task-relevant skill can serve as a predominant basis of treating and recognizing individuals if its importance is made clear to group progress. If task-relevant skill is not emphasized, then social hierarchies and biases often seep into and end up structuring interaction.

We do not view people as fully unique. Instead, we view them in terms of their class, gender, race, age, ability, marital status, and other social categories. Typically, gender is one of the first things we assume or notice when meeting someone new—we are "framed before we know it" into gender identities that bias interpretations of our behavior (Ridgeway 2009, 2011)—along with race, age, and social class. We are far from neutral in our first impressions of others and the trajectories along which social interaction proceeds (Ridgeway 2014). Communication and motivation follow from assumptions and expectations, which in turn follow from social categorizations and roles. In fact, we might even understand this fractional treatment of each other as the structural indignity of enduring society as an individual person.

These status characteristics, and others, are socially constructed and go on to shape social interactions in ways that, on average, tend to reinforce the existing power hierarchies of those same societies. Indeed, status attached to social categories tracks historically with wealth and influence attached to these same categories. In *The Source of Self-Regard*, Toni Morrison (2019) follows many social and economic historians in conceptualizing wealth—across the generations and centuries—as a transhistorical and intergenerational financialization of violence. Wealth carries its origins in property and situation, and property and situation either are inherited and thus resist social upheaval through intergenerational persistence or are appropriated through structural or physical violence. At the micro level, this leads to status beliefs about the members of groups. The past resource levels of the categories we fall into shape how we are perceived as individuals within those groups today.

By extension, demographic groups—defined by gender, race, or age, for example—that historically have enjoyed more power, prestige, or status tend to do so in the future due to how we interact with these groups in ways that implicitly acknowledge these social histories. These observed treatments involve subtle status signals that our brains notice: body language, verbal dominance, and vocal inflection all register as signals of hierarchical standing. For instance, these conversational inequalities (Cannon, Robinson, and Smith-Lovin 2019) can involve being interrupted early in a social interaction, leading to cumulative disadvantage for the remainder of a conversation. Audit studies in sociology and economics uncover persistent disadvantages by race, gender, or age in whether individuals are hired or perceived as competent (Grusky and Hill 2018).

The coexistence of persistent social inequality with lowered rates of explicit or acknowledged bias (e.g., Hunt et al. 2013; Hunt, Croll, and Krysan 2022) raises all kinds of complicated questions about how status hierarchies might continue to exist. To a large degree, they will perpetuate because of external structures such as social institutions, which we touch on in more depth in Chapter 4. To help us see how this could happen at the individual level, however, the Stanford sociologist Cecilia Ridgeway (2011, 2019) draws on multiple, eminent programs of status characteristics research evidence to argue that "third-order beliefs"—what *we* believe *most people* believe about age, gender, race, profession, education, or any other status—contribute to the social elevation of categories above the people who occupy and live within them. In other words, an expectation that men or white people will be viewed as more competent by most people in the context of decision-making or performance is powerful enough to uphold a status hierarchy, even while individuals themselves may not be or see themselves as prejudiced at all. Many explicit or clear forms of prejudice or bigotry have "moved underground." Racism does not need racists, only structures, interactions, and expectations that end up privileging by race—even if this is not the anticipated outcome or the desired outcome (Bonilla-Silva 2010).

Moreover, internalized self-beliefs can reinforce status characteristics: they lead to biased self-assessments (Correll 2001). For instance, internalized ageism results in the premature aging of adults, as individuals feel pessimistic about their ability to age well (Levy et al. 2009). Moreover, internalized gender biases about science and math lead women, on average, to feel less confident than men at the same objective ability levels (Correll 2001).

Other status-based viewpoints on dignity focus on culture broadly understood. Nietzsche saw dignity in terms of aesthetics. Art, he recognized, originated from the exploitation of the labor of nonartists to produce the space and leisure necessary for its "proper" conception and execution. In other words, Nietzsche came full circle in conceptualizing dignity as high art consumed by a select few, supposedly unappreciated by the uncultured, its elite production enabled by mass indignities of calcified social inequalities. Bourdieu (1984) similarly discussed how elites distinguish themselves by creating and preferring distinctive art forms. By extension, a culture in which high art is valorized is itself rife with indignity and hierarchy, which could inform debates about how indignity is both the basis and subject of commercially successful art.

Regardless, the point remains: current dignities hardly are isolated from past indignities toward others, and the dehumanizing effects of past indignities linger across time and history. One of the modern tragedies of social existence is that we are socialized to support hierarchies even if we personally object to them. We are socialized to believe that status is proof of value, and we tend to act in ways that perpetuate status by assigning worth to status. Age stereotypes, gender stereotypes, and racial or ethnic categorizations all are based in hierarchies of worth, in a culture where men hold wealth and power, where youth is valorized, and where institutions are historically white dominated.

Our identity,[10] and therefore our beliefs about what justice looks like, follow from the statuses that individuals hold (Hegtvedt 2006; McLeod, Hallett, and Lively 2015; Schnittker and McLeod 2005; Schwalbe et al. 2000). Thus, dignity shapes and reflects the ways in which status, identity, and justice are enacted in any specific society (Roscigno, Yavorsky, and Quadlin 2021).

## Human Dignity as Supersession of Status and Hierarchy

Each of us must endure society in order to stay a part of it, because personhood gains meaning only with—only through—the socially defined identities and categories that make us who we are. Given what we know about how status works in society, calls for dignity seem to be attempts to frame a shared humanity to supersede and rewrite these categories and, as such, to reconstruct their associated social meanings and valuations, as Simmel imagined when referring to humanity as a master status (see Hodgkiss 2018).

---

[10] A term perhaps as loaded as dignity; see Burke and Stets (2009) for one extensive treatment, and Owens, Smith-Lovin, and Robinson (2010) for a broader view; see Brubaker and Cooper (2000) for a skeptical account of the term.

"The particularistic rights of status groups and of circles are replaced in prin-ciple by the rights of the individual, and these, quite significantly, are called 'human rights'; that is, they are the rights that derive from belonging to the widest conceivable circle," Georg Simmel (2012, 379) said.

Recent violence has elicited viral social reminders—often disheartened pleas—that #BlackLivesMatter, countered by #AllLivesMatter and conversations about privilege and inequality in America. Recently, Asian American students marched around the university campuses nationwide, holding signs proclaiming "#Iamnotavirus" and "#stopasianhate." Other viral calls for accountability, such as #metoo and #timesup, call for more dig-nity in the workplace and a cessation of workplace harassment and abuse.

What do social justice hashtags have in common? They seem to be more than just calls for safety. They are proclamations about what individuals should reasonably expect from society, and how those expectations entangle with the categories in which individuals find themselves.

## Dignity as Social Endurance: Preserving, Creating, and Defining Individuality against Social Violence

As we face life, we endure what it brings from the locations in which we find ourselves, physically and socially. That is, being an individual involves a per-sonal standpoint as well as a social location. By virtue of how we are differ-ently classed, racialized, gendered, or resourced, and socialized within and across our social categories, we all have emergent, novel standpoints and ex-perienced flows of time and future horizons (Emirbayer and Mische 1998; Hitlin 2008) by which we interpret ourselves and the world.

We all face challenges and difficulties. However, on balance, it is well es-tablished that stresses at the top of social hierarchies have a far lesser im-pact on health, disease, and early death in the aggregate than do markers of strain, humiliation, disadvantage, or risky environmental exposures in lower socioeconomic strata. These inequalities in stress produce the well-known gradients in population health by socioeconomic status as famously published by Sir Michael Marmot in the 1990s (Siegrist and Marmot 2004). Health psychologist Nancy Adler and medical sociologist Bruce Link con-tinue to review evidence from dozens of national and international datasets that one's higher position within and across social hierarchies bears a funda-mental relationship to one's health and longevity. Stress is a part of life, but stress among the disadvantaged is much more harmful to health and overall life expectancy.

The subjective nature of these objective difficulties varies. People interpret their lives in terms of having to endure various difficulties to become or to remain who they think they are or should be. Many life narratives involve some perseverance, or overcoming, of some kind of perceived obstacle. Perhaps the royal family feels they have had an easy time of it, but even they discuss the travails of being wealthy and representing a country; increasingly, celebrities are sharing their personal health struggles with the world, such as Justin Bieber's public disclosure of facial paralysis following Hailey Bieber's vlogging of her transient ischemic attack (mini stroke).[11]

So, what does each of us endure biologically and socially, and what do we perceive that we *should* endure—on any given day or in the long term? An often-suggested path to dignity lies through asserting one's endurance in the face of these difficulties.[12] We argue that subjective dignity can be understood as an indicator of what individuals perceive themselves as enduring, measured within their own minds against what they believe they should endure.

The social conditions of endurance are inseparable from personalized understandings of what it means to be the person one is. Personhood occurs across and between—not within—roles, identities, selves, values, and beliefs. As many scholars have pointed out, there is dignity in striving and suffering, provided it is struggle or growth arcing toward perceived acceptance, purpose, or recognition despite social adversities. Meanwhile, of course, structural indignities exist whether or not we perceive them, as noted in Karl Marx's concept of false consciousness and by sociological scholars of structural injustice beginning with W. E. B. DuBois.

Clearly, some significant, ongoing level of individual social endurance is fundamental to becoming a person and to having and maintaining dignity. But how much? And when does it become too much? If dignity is about what we put up with in exchange for what we want, then what is the role of projection or imagination into the future (Mische 2009)?

Nobody deserves to be mistreated, but how we understand mistreatment and its remediation are likely to be vital to the experience of dignity. This pertains especially in lives where misfortune, abuse, and marginalization are

---

[11] "Justin Bieber is one of many stars sharing personal health struggles," *Washington Post*, June 12, 2022.

[12] The rise and fall of the psychological notion of "grit" (Duckworth et al. 2007) displays this sort of mindset. For one review, see Kwon 2017.

abundant. Across multiple hierarchies defined by status, we all experience degrees of privilege and marginalization. Through optimism and a sense of mastery or competence, individuals might partly sustain their dignities in the present (e.g., Frye 2012). For instance, optimism in America rests on a presumed ability to better oneself through hard work or through opportunity.

By extension, if individuals find themselves unable to imagine something resembling a desirable future for themselves, then dignity perhaps first involves trying to break free of oppressions or contexts that stifle the will or imagination. If one dies while held in the grasp of overwhelming oppressions, or without a perceived bright future, then dignity might be about how one weathered and approached one's suffering as best one could, given one's oppressive situation within the world.

# 3

# Beyond Reason

## Finding Dignity in Social Relations

In the preceding two chapters, we first organized diverse conceptual perspectives on dignity and then provided a rationale for treating dignity as a public health issue. In this chapter, we build on these definitional and public health approaches to dignity by explaining how dignity is rooted in social relations—and thus is transmitted and learned through acts of care or neglect.

We may at root be self-interested beings, but a lot of scientific evidence suggests we also are compassionate and that connecting with others is a basis of learning and survival. Here, we develop a more detailed perspective on how dignity seems to work in actual social relations between people. In doing so, we focus on the practical and moral basis of dignity: what dignity might look like and what it means as we find out and express who we are as individuals through social relationships.

Morality, understood both scientifically and classically, is less about a prescriptive recipe for living a good life and more about the study of social life (Hitlin 2021; Parish 2014). Durkheim saw sociology as the study of moral life, the essence of being a social species needing to coordinate action among self-interested members of a society. He originally wanted to name sociology as some version of "moral-ology" (Abend 2008). Morality is about what organizes individuals into predictable action.

We distinguish emotion and care from "pure rationality" to make the point that dignity—like morality itself—reflects experiences of care or neglect, which defy strictly rational explanation or proof.[1] We have different logics or ways of talking about how people ought to be or how they ought to act (Lamont and Thévenot 2000). While we might be more likely to pursue

---

[1] Empirical psychological science finds that one cannot, in the practice of human minds, so neatly distinguish emotion and rationality (e.g., Damasio 1994), but the theoretical cleavage allows us purchase to more precisely focus on the emotional experience of dignity.

*The Science of Dignity.* Steven Hitlin and Matthew A. Andersson, Oxford University Press.
© Oxford University Press 2023. DOI: 10.1093/oso/9780197743867.003.0004

actions for which legitimate explanations exist (Mills 1940; Gerth and Mills 1953), possible actions are so numerous that morality becomes vital for explaining how people select from various possible behaviors or justifications for those behaviors. "Reason is, in fact, both the ally and the enemy of dignity," Philip Hodgkiss (2018, 155) once quipped.

When National Institutes of Health (NIH) director Dr. Anthony Fauci lamented, "I don't know how to explain to you that you should care for other people," he was referring to the fact that caring is an individual behavior and yet also a set of moral intuitions we learn from the societies and institutions guiding us. He also seemed to be expressing some frustration at how discussions of caring or protection start from different assumptions about how individuals and societies ought to relate—and how these assumptions in many ways exist beyond the realm of logical debate. If they exist before logic, then they find their origins in social relationships, and in how those relationships lead to differing practical orientations to human dignity.

## Looking for Dignity in the Origins of Social Order

Social order—seen as patterned regularities in behavior—is necessary for the safety and continued existence of individuals in a social environment. This lack of order is terrifying. Ten concertgoers died at the rapper Travis Scott's Astroworld Festival in Houston, Texas, in December 2021, when an intentionally rowdy crowd trapped individuals to the point of suffocation. The security manual for Astroworld did "not discuss anything significant about what to do in an emergency situation" even though Scott often encourages unruly audiences. According to the same manual, any "dead" or "deceased" concertgoers were to be referred to as "smurf[s]" so that the show could, it would seem, go on.[2]

Rosen (2012) remarks that "self-regarding duties set limits to our freedom" (148). These self-regarding duties, as it turns out, are society-regarding or society-disregarding duties.[3] Existential freedom—you can jump up and

[2] "Astroworld's Safety Plan Called for Deceased to Be Referred to as 'Smurfs,'" NPR National News, November 10, 2021. Soon after the news of these concert-driven deaths by suffocation, the public drew a sharp contrast between Scott's concert and Adele's one decade earlier, when she halted the show to provide urgent help to one fan who had fainted.

[3] James Coleman (1988), Nan Lin (2002), and other scholars of social capital have long recognized that community networks represent, at their core, a coordination and maintenance problem. Namely, they are established and maintained only in the presence of an individual will toward collective investment anchored in mutual trust and norms of reciprocity.

sing show tunes anywhere, technically speaking—is practically trivial much of the time (Hitlin and Elder 2007), even if still of conceptual interest to philosophers like Sartre.[4]

How, exactly, do individuals and societies relate in a way that preserves both types of entities? Similarly, what exactly does it mean *socially* to have an *individual* body and mind? Is this the same thing as having freedom? Our Gallup dignity data were collected before and during the Covid-19 pandemic, a worldwide event that prodded at social orders we took for granted. As such, while a collective tragedy, it also is an opportunity to probe some basic questions about the nature of order, individuals, and their complicated relationship, as indicated by the senses of dignity.

Somewhat recently, we contributed to an edited book entitled *Order on the Edge of Chaos* (Lawler, Thye, and Yoon 2015). Its purpose was to collect perspectives on how social order originates and is maintained. We offered dignity as a link between individuality and society. *We argued that because people are motivated to achieve and maintain dignity as individuals, they maintain local as well as broader forms of social order as a byproduct of their actions.* A key conceptual issue for understanding dignity is appreciating how local social orders can differ noticeably from broader or societal orders that enfold higher levels of structure, such as in the context of segregation or polarization.

Dignity, we wrote, is at root a motivation for and a practice of "social personhood": people are "persons" who use society to understand themselves and others (e.g., Cahill 1998; Smith 2009). Dignity presupposes collective social life, and thus smuggles in aspects of mutual recognition and concern, even if the ultimate desired end is "pure" individual rights.[5] Dignity exists somehow outside of human interaction; at the same time, dignity is an achievement that is fundamentally interpersonal and personal.

In many applications, dignity involves autonomy, nonhumiliation, and the realization of social purposes as they are locally defined (Callero 2018; Habermas 2010; Hodson 2001; Lamont 2000; Misztal 2013).

As the sociologist Andrew Sayer notes, to analyze dignity is to analyze the very essence of "our deeply social nature." Dignity is recognized and realized "only in actual relations" and "evident only in the concreteness of human life and practice" (Malpas and Lickiss 2007, 5). Human beings are relational

[4] Sartre later toned down his extreme focus on individual freedom in service of acknowledging the power of social life as necessary for human social existence.
[5] This recalls our key point in Chapter 1 about the socially constructed nature of autonomy.

(e.g., Emirbayer and Goodwin 1994), given how their selves are culturally and linguistically mediated, "exist[ing] only within webs of interlocution" (Taylor 1992) and are born of, not prior to, socialization. While a mythos of self-sufficiency might suggest otherwise, people are reciprocally influential. Who we "are" only makes sense within or against a web of social ties or commitments (Taylor 1991, 1992). Our life projects, in Archer's (2007) terms, involve taking stands on issues. Even by taking no stand at all, we are positioning ourselves symbolically on the sidelines.

Morality reflects background social expectations (e.g., Abend 2013) that frame experiences of self-worth in the perceived eyes of others. Dignity embodies "proper moves" within a socially defined game, where the game itself is defined by those with whom one plays, to paraphrase Pierre Bourdieu's perspective on social practice. Having a feel for the game involves internalizing the rules, roles, and standards for various situations. As such, dignity is about situated morality; morality can involve tradeoffs across moments, such as committing what is viewed as grave wrongdoing in the service of social conformity (e.g., "I was just following orders or doing what I was told to do").[6] To be a human is to live with moral perspectives ("horizons," in Taylor's parlance) through which we judge the world and make attributions of good or bad, even if only within our own minds. And those perspectives come to us as possibilities we both understand and debate, through our families, friends, schools, and other institutions that exist within a wider, societal set of cultural beliefs.

Because it spans time and biography, dignity is prone to contradictions (Emirbayer and Mische 1998; Hitlin and Elder 2007; Sanchez, Lamont, and Zilberstein 2022). For instance, in *Remaking a Life*, Celeste Watkins-Hayes (2019) often refers to the dignity that individuals living with stigma manage to achieve, in terms of how individuals make the journey from "dying from" to "living with" HIV or AIDS (see also Watkins-Hayes, Pittman-Gay, and Beaman 2012). Their transformative projects, as she calls them, are reflective of agency, and this agency works through specialized health and community organizations that restructure their finances, their social networks, their community engagement, and their approach to disease management.

---

[6] Todd May (2017) and other philosophers have warned of the false logic inherent in historical counterfactuals. It is entirely possible that, without atrocities, perhaps especially World War II, the Universal Declaration of Human Rights would not have received its particular impetus or historic importance. Elements of history only make sense in the context of each other, a quandary we cannot hope to sort out here.

Through these multiple avenues, individuals achieve a sense of dignity by seeing a life past their diagnosis and enlarging their identities beyond the social stigma ascribed to AIDS.

## Called to Order: Thinking about Care in the Context of Recent Social Chaos

Bellah and colleagues (1985) discussed how collectively oriented action is ultimately an individual choice. Lichterman (1995) refers to this as the "seesaw" model, the idea that people must balance individual gain with helping others. Empirically, some people do see the world this way, but many see these two supposed polarities as complementary (Hitlin and Salisbury 2013). This does not mean that people who are vaccine hesitant or vaccine opposed are not caring: it means that how they care for themselves and others depends on their understandings of what care looks like.

Consider how just 1.7% of Papua New Guineans were vaccinated against Covid-19. As Fraser Macdonald explains, the extreme vaccine situation in Papua New Guinea hardly reflects access or rollout: instead, it reflects an opposition based in a cultural context where biomedical explanations of disease are viewed as secondary to spiritual explanations, and where vaccines therefore represent a fundamental threat to existing culture.[7] Caring involves putting spirit before body.

In the United States, vaccine hesitancy is understood in terms of perceptions of risk and in terms of partisan or religious background, and in some geographic areas in terms of access or rollout. People are attempting to take care of themselves in ways that make sense to them, and the results for nationwide pandemic mortality and spread can be disastrous. In areas with increased spread, partisan divide over the Covid response might become slightly more muted (Rodriguez et al. 2022), speaking to a limited power of firsthand encounters with death for reducing political polarization. The pandemic also could reflect a fraying relationship between individuals and their societies, born of mistrust or skepticism about what society or its institutions can offer them, what Tom Nichols (2017) positioned within a broader trend in the digital world: the "death of (formal) expertise."

[7] Fraser Macdonald, "Just 1.7% of People in PNG Are Vaccinated against COVID. Why Is Resistance So Fierce?," *The Conversation*, November 7, 2021.

We can debate how caring individuals are, as psychological research into empathy and altruism has facilitated (see Piliavin 2008 for one review). Sociologically speaking, we only hear people's reports of their own motivations (Mills 1940; Vaisey 2009), and thus we can analyze the cultural logics people use when talking about how and why they care for others. A logic of care among those who are vaccine hesitant might involve managing perceived risks to themselves or significant others, along with a sense that scientific or governmental elites are wrong or have vested or undisclosed interests, or an emphasis on the fact that the vaccine is "only approved for emergency use," or on the fact that one is not personally old or medically vulnerable.

How individuals approach and prioritize these different types of harm seems terribly relevant to both individual and collective dignity during the pandemic. Clearly, caring involves a differentiation of types of potential harm, who might be harmed, and how badly. Plenty of moral outrage has resulted: for instance, some have cast vaccine-hesitant individuals as extremely selfish or as unwilling to make even the smallest sacrifice for others. According to a recent *New Yorker* cartoon, beekeepers might decline protective gear because of their "rights," but this does not change the external risks. Swarms of bees might represent more of a clear and present danger, perhaps, but our need to ensure our own safety and that of others is a constant one in life and one that can be a source of anger, grief, or profound tragedy.

When Ohio representative Jim Jordan referred to vaccine mandates as "un-American," he was drawing on a particular understanding ("logic") of what it might mean to be American, centered on a rugged individualism even at the expense of a collective good. In a *Washington Post* response, Americanism was portrayed in terms of George Washington's requirement for his troops to be immunized, and the similar decisions made by presidents and military leaders.[8] Drawing an artificial distinction between Americanism as an individual ideal and Americanism as a shared, collective quest can lead to opposing understandings of what it means to care: caring for oneself can be presented either as a way of resisting coercion or as a way of caring for others.

Adam Smith based his famous economic treatises on the fact that humans possess "sympathy"; in his work, the "invisible hand" only makes sense if

---

[8] Timothy Bella, "Jim Jordan Says Vaccine Mandates Are Un-American. George Washington Thought Otherwise," *Washington Post*, September 7, 2021.

humans have a caring for others that curbs economic exploitation naturally.[9] Few people extend their circles of care about others indiscriminately; a lot of research shows that care exists more easily within close relations. In many cases, it coldly dissipates when confronted with outsiders whom we perceive to be unlike ourselves (e.g., Berreby 2005; Greene 2013). Just as we are more caring toward those in our inner circles, we are more moved to action by their experiences. Restricting care to close others does not mean we have forgotten how to care more broadly. Yet, how widely we extend feelings of care is a social issue, one that is dynamic and subject to change.

How we care depends on how we draw boundaries between ourselves and outsiders and if we define some of them as our enemies. This can become a political project: former Afghanistan president Hamid Karzai formed a coordinating council soon after the Taliban invasion, "to prevent chaos and reduce the suffering of the people."[10] Ukrainian president Volodymyr Zelenskyy mobilized his people in the fight against Russia. Pandemic research has shown how close contact with a Covid case is linked to an increased probability of engaging in protective behaviors such as social distancing or masking.[11]

## Getting Subjective: Seeing the Social in the Personal

Sociology decenters the person from explanations of what is possible or probable. People make sense of who they are, and who they might become, based on what is happening to the people around them (Elder 1994).[12] There

[9] One might suggest Smith missed the boat on very real possibilities for social violence and exploitation, also endemic in humans. Oddly, economists spend a lot of time on *The Wealth of Nations* and not very much on *The Moral Sentiments*, his companion work. The infamous "invisible hand" that motivates so much of free market ideology only made sense, to Smith, if people were, in fact, sympathetic to each other.

[10] "The Taliban Tighten Their Grip on Kabul as Afghanistan's Government Disintegrates," NPR, August 15, 2021.

[11] "Adults with Close Contacts That Tested Positive for COVID Are More Likely to Restrict Their Daily Behaviors Due to COVID-19," press release, Longitudinal Study of Dynamics of Social Life during COVID-19, Department of Sociology, Yale University, https://campuspress.yale.edu/dslco vid/fact-sheet-3/, accessed August 20, 2021.

[12] Though we operate in a wider world of institutions and distant forces, much of our lives comes down to our intimate groups and relationships, what Cooley (1902) referred to as our primary groups. In order for an abstract concept like dignity to have a role in human motivation, it would need to function similarly to a relational schema—a mental construct woven from concrete interpersonal histories and their emotional moments (Cerulo 2010). This means we cognitively internalize a sense of what someone else would do in a situation one is encountering, of a possible self or ideal self that is socialized from one's significant others, reference groups, or "circle of recognition" more broadly (Andersen and Chen 2002; Berger and Luckmann 1966).

is no personal understanding without social understanding. The personal fundamentally reflects the social, what John Levi Martin (2001) called the "sociological hunch."

People's actions are shaped to a considerable degree by external forces. At the same time, people make choices: they have what is termed "agency," and this agency is bounded by historical, material, and social circumstances (Emirbayer and Mische 1998; Hitlin and Johnson 2015; Shanahan and Hood 2000). As Marx famously wrote: "Men [sic] make their own history, but they do not make it as they please; they do not make it under self-selected circumstances, but under circumstances existing already, given and transmitted from the past."[13] Historical and structural inequalities shape and constrain routes toward personal destinies.

The sociologist C. Wright Mills (1959) articulated the "sociological imagination" when he stated: "The individual can understand her own experience and gauge her own fate only by locating herself within her period, that she can know her own chances in life only by becoming aware of those of all individuals in her circumstances." While Mills is right that individual experience rests on the social understandings that individuals have about their positions in society, these understandings take shape across multiple levels of social reality. Individuals experience social institutions, such as a family, a government, a school, or a workplace, in terms of their specific place within them (Berger and Luckmann 1966). To people, social institutions exude a humbling sense of being larger than any specific relationship, because of their perceived independent legitimacy. This legitimacy has an undercurrent of morality, captured in Goffman's (1983) notion of the "moral order" (see Rawls and McMurrin 1987; Rawls 1999). Relationships between two individuals take a micro-institutional form, in the sense of a third, independent entity—a social bond—creating ritual and regularity between two autonomous individuals (Berger and Luckmann 1966). Violating these regularities (e.g., Garfinkel 1967) leads to emotional reactions and sometimes to social sanctions. People are expected to act or contribute in structured ways that acknowledge social order while reflecting individuality.

The sociologist Dennis Wrong (1961) wrote, following Sigmund Freud, that humans are "social, asocial, and antisocial." Dignity, we suggest, integrates all three realities: dignity is socially fragile or given, intrinsic to

---

[13] He goes on to say: "The tradition of all dead generations weighs like a nightmare on the brains of the living." Marx was a tad less optimistic than we are about society's potential.

humankind and thus asocial or biological, and sometimes maintained "antisocially" by bucking or restructuring society as with different forms of social protest. Self-knowledge depends on, and is impossible without, knowledge of others, or the world more generally. This is the epistemic relationality of dignity: "a sense of dignity due to a sense of worth in relation to ourselves" that arises in our relation to others and the world itself. Further, "dignity that belongs to a human life . . . refers us instead to the worth of a human life which is given only through the articulation of that life in relation to self, other, and world" (Malpas 2007, 24).

George H. Mead's (1934) theory of reflected appraisals states that we learn to think about ourselves based on how we imagine others think about us, all of which takes place through symbolic material such as culture and language. As children, we rehearse this process, and as adults, we take it for granted. How we relate to ourselves is itself an internalization of how significant others early in our lives relate to us, and the words, objects, and gestures they present, use, and value.[14] Similarly, the dignity philosopher Stephen Darwall referred to the immediacy of "second-personal" experience, whether in person or online (Campos-Castillo and Hitlin 2013; Shilling and Mellor 2022).[15] Through attachment to others, we simultaneously transcend ourselves and create ourselves. Self-construction is self-destruction, in that creating a self means decimating certain possibilities or potentialities that will not come to be, at least not in the foreseeable future.[16]

Our social circles, in turn, are influenced by broader cultures. Ann Swidler recently described culture as providing "theories of self," and in this sense culture provides dignity as a moral tool for understanding how a self might be enacted and experienced. Self-disapproval might mean that one seeks a dignity they feel missing. For instance, individuals might look at their lives and have a difficult time deciding what counts as "selflessness" or "selfishness," and why. To resolve these complex moral deliberations, individuals can turn to a more holistic approach,[17] in which they imagine *who* they are becoming across all their roles and commitments in society; in order

---

[14] See Franks (2010) on one early interpretation of these links, but see Firat and Hitlin (2012) on a mild critique. Abrutyn and Lizardo (2020) link these insights with some of what we know about neurological processes.

[15] Engels' point that the I-thou bond is spiritual if not transcendent sounds a similar note; Martin Buber makes the same general conceptual point as well.

[16] This would be an understudied flipside to Markus and Nurius' (1986) notion of "possible selves."

[17] Many (e.g., Thoits 1983) demonstrate that holding more roles in society is associated with better mental health through providing more opportunities to construct, and buffer, a positive vision of oneself.

to imagine who they are becoming, they refer to a self that has been—and is being—created from relationships with others and continues to operate meaningfully or intelligibly only with reference to this situated, in-progress self (Emirbayer 1997; Mead 1934; Gerth and Mills 1953).[18] The focus of much social science research is on specific, self-related processes like "self-esteem," "self-enhancement," the "moral self," or "identity."[19] Less focus has been on whether these motivations may be part of an overarching social personhood or individuality, one guided by broader moral principles or some sense of coherence across all these disparate psychological systems.

Goffman raised the issue of the "person and her collaborative manufacture" as central to social interaction (Cahill 1998). Persons are embedded in bodies and given selves continually by and through society. Following Hegel, "man is recognized and treated as a rational being, as free, as a person; and the individual, on his side, makes himself worthy of this recognition by overcoming the natural state of his self-consciousness and obeying a universal. . . . [H]e behaves, therefore, towards others in a manner that is universally valid, recognizing them—as he wishes others to recognize him—as free, as persons" (Douzinas 2002, 388). Consider the sociologist Pierre Bourdieu's (1990, 15) provocative suggestion that "sociology frees us from the illusion of freedom, or, more exactly from the misplaced belief in illusory freedoms." At the same time, the study of psychology would make little sense if people did not experience themselves as somehow free and distinct from others and from society, and people with the same social location do not behave identically.

Is there a way to maintain the holistic and authentic nature of a person— we do not experience ourselves as simply a conglomeration of components, variables, or dispositions—while also studying them scientifically? The idea of "self" is inferred socially from personhood, not the other way around, making self a "secondary and derivative reality" that others enable us to have by relating to us in a way that suggests we are unique or worthy in our own right (Cahill 1998). The social manufacture of a self is one of "joint ceremonial labor" in which individuals are given room to be the particular people

---

[18] Agentic beliefs are socially constructed in terms of the types of individuals people believe they can become based on where they are and the resources and capacities they possess. While Bellah and colleagues (1985) outline "therapist" and "manager" types, Riesman, Glazer, and Denney (2020) outline "inner-directed" and "outer-directed" individuals; these archetypal visions stem from deeper conceptions about legitimate self-constructions that exist beyond, but are informed by, particular habits or values.

[19] See Tesser et al. (2000) on the "self-zoo."

they are. Names and appearances further substantiate the existences of selves.[20]

## Dignity as the Creative Cocreation of Individuality and Society

There are ways to neglect individuality when understanding society,[21] such as focusing on gender or race as the sole factor explaining behavior across all situations. Sociologists save themselves from these sorts of reductionisms in at least two important ways. First, they analyze individuals at the intersection of multiple contexts and identities, rarely presuming that individual action is sufficiently dictated by a single factor. Second, sociologists appeal to agency or context to understand why even some of the best statistical models predict far less than a quarter of all observed differences within a key outcome measure like income, happiness, or health.

Creativity is the possibility to do differently or act unexpectedly, for better or for worse. Humans lead patterned lives, but much variation in the world comes from individual choices and, more importantly, the sheer uniqueness of each social situation. In fact, individuals exhibit creativity even in routine situations (e.g., Joas 2000), having to adjust within the moment to interaction partners. We do not know exactly what we and others will do, even in situations we have been in hundreds of times, like driving to work, picking up the kids, or going to a ballgame. In-the-moment creativity is necessary for successful, sustained social interaction. Anybody might drop their drink, forget a name, or say something unexpected. We can stop and stare, or we can move the situation along.

We need to handle situations with some tact; otherwise we risk impairing our dignity and that of others (Goffman 1963). If we treat each other too automatically or without enough attention to the situation unfolding, we risk being labeled as unfeeling, callous, or robotic, all of which suggest that we are

---

[20] Laws, rights, or ceremonies as social realities underwriting personhood are separate from the "actual occasions of social interaction" or "interpretive frameworks of accountability" that are brought to bear in the realization of persons (Cahill 1998).

[21] For a review of Parsons' work and its pushback along this interpretation, see Joas and Knobl (2009). Also noteworthy is Garfinkel's critique of the idea that macrosociology turns people into "cultural dopes" (e.g., Granovetter 1985). Donald Black (2002) has tried to advance a "pure sociology," attached even to morality, that focuses on patterns moving people through society without any need to focus on those people.

acting in a subhuman, undignified way in the dramaturgy of life. To be human is to be creative within role-related constraints: that is, to be adequately creative within moments based on situational demands and obligations. While individuals might disagree about what authenticity or individuality ought to look like, individuals still intuitively appreciate a sense of (in)authenticity as a social interaction unfolds.

Perhaps, then, a vital misunderstanding of dignity would involve overlooking the thoroughly creative nature of social life. Sociologist Hans Joas posits that capitalism has largely succeeded in marginalizing the perceived domain of creativity to the realms of the avant-garde and the eccentric geniuses, darkly fulfilling what Marx saw as a growing chasm between true work and repetitive labor. "Regular" creativity—the kind that happens or ought to happen in hobbies, friendships, work, romantic relationships, business transactions, or grocery store conversations—is underplayed, and only professional versions of Creativity valorized by cultural institutions, such as music or art, are popularly recognized as "creative." This narrow or conventional view on creativity is a huge mistake, we think, when it comes to understanding how individuals thoughtfully maintain or neglect each other's dignity as well as different, larger types of social order.

One of Joas' broader points about creativity is that it is a metaphor for life itself, one that breaks free of animalistic visions of stimulus-response and normativized visions of "cultural dopes" who enact roles without a meaningful semblance of individuality. That is, Joas draws attention to what Turner (1978) might have called "role-distancing" in the service of individual agency. Without sufficient creativity in defining or navigating one's circumstances, a slow sense of alienation develops. To feel alive, for some,[22] is to actively choose for oneself in combinations that never have been chosen together before.

To be clear, much social behavior is habitual or routine in nature and therefore does not directly implicate a sense of self or identity (Gecas 2003) much less any values at the self's core (e.g., Hitlin 2003). The self only matters some of the time, but those are often the most subjectively or emotionally memorable junctures of one's days and one's life. Much of the time we are simply living in line with habits (Camic 1986) or social expectations (Hitlin and

---

[22] Ralph Turner (1976) discussed different aspects of the "real self" and found (Turner and Schutte 1981) that some people feel real in moments of freedom, while others feel that way when filling social roles and expectations.

Elder 2007). However, even during these moments, personal identity is evident as individual, creative action or "expressive identifiability" (Goffman 1974): how one speaks, what one wears, how one moves, how one laughs or expresses concern, anger, or care.

Maintaining an expected or desired presentation of self is attached to one's subjective sense of dignity. Dignity stems from an "authentic morality" (Joas 1996, 258), which "integrates meaningfully into the personal balance of a meaningful life." Subjective dignity might be felt when or as "the openness of self-articulation is wedded to the responsibility of self-control" (255), in which life resists anomic "aestheticization" associated with postmodernism and instead confronts the inherent tensions of normativity and living a personally satisfying moral life.[23] We "distance ourselves from morality" as strictly prescriptive, while morality itself distances us from destructive tendencies within each of us (258).

## Toward a Pragmatic Perspective on Dignity

In the fiftieth anniversary edition of *Interaction of Color*, the master artist and teacher Josef Albers (2013) provides a variety of exhibits that demonstrate that human vision sees color not in any absolute sense, but rather as a visual effect.

To help us understand how this works, Albers first advances the notion of a "factual fact," or what he defines in terms of wavelengths or other physical properties of light.[24] He then sharply contrasts the "factual facts" of colors with "practical" considerations that are called "actual facts": "But when we see opaque color as transparent or perceive opacity as translucence . . . when we see 3 colors as 4 or as 2 . . . [t]hese effects we call actual facts," he writes.

By equating the actual with the practical, Albers provides a way of thinking about how William James, Hans Joas, Neil Gross, and others have defined social pragmatism: *thinking is for acting, or is always oriented around social actions taken, perceived, or imagined.*

---

[23] We might suggest that people satisfice their morality (Gigerenzer 2010; Hitlin 2008) by doing enough to feel morally adequate, if not striving to live like moral exemplars.

[24] Note that factual facts themselves are based in what Albers calls "acknowledged" systems of measurement, in the same way that the quantum physicist Werner Heisenberg defines science in terms of choice of method. This implies that colors could factually exist in manners other than wavelength, as measurement systems are themselves based in theory.

Dignity exists in this pragmatic spirit: it does not and never has existed in a vacuum. A pragmatic approach to dignity helps us understand how dignity is a matter of solving social problems in the moment. It also helps us understand why dignity is hard to define in any absolute sense, and why so much of dignity rests on how individuals understand the situation they are in. Hodgkiss (2018) puts this correctly when he traces dignity to "perceiving the imperceptible."

*When, how, and why* we do what we do inflects any interpersonal perception of *what* we do, in a way that makes real and meaningful sense to the individuals who are involved. People experience right and wrong intuitively, not as a calculus. We are often more logical after the fact than we were in the moment of action (e.g., Vaisey 2009). After the fact, people sometimes attempt to pass justifications for actions that might feel deceitful, callous, or audacious to those who are involved in a situation.

Human cognition evolved to solve problems in the physical world. We have abstracted that capacity to remarkable lengths, but just as babies make sense of their world physically before they have language, humans think about the world first as a way to solve immediate problems in their physical—then later social—environments. Survival is the ultimate practical concern, and other concerns are all practical as well, in the sense of relating to social practice in some form.

If human thinking itself is oriented or made possible by practical realities including goals, relationships, and language, then what does this mean for the "true essence" of ourselves, others, or the world itself? Such an essence may be a social construction, and as such, can dignity be said to have any "true essence"? Here again, the logic of Albers' color study is relevant: colors are perceived through larger visual contexts, just as selves are made and then perceived through larger social contexts. Social contexts shape problems we face and need to solve; our senses of self—of who we *are*—develop along the way.

Yet, we also have some sense of ourselves independent of the situation we currently are in. We experience ourselves as distinct from our social surroundings, even if we are not fully distinct. Some essentialisms—that is, static, definable, or discrete entities—are necessary for living in society and for the operation of scientific inquiry. Harrison White (1992) and others have pointed out that social science essentialisms may be misappropriations of essentialist concepts from the natural sciences. Casting individuals as discrete agents, for example, facilitates many forms of statistical analysis and social science theory generation. The natural sciences use chemistry and physics to make sense of the essentials of life: atoms are not, in verifiable fact, the discrete, didactic spheres of textbooks, nor is it even clear what they tangibly represent in any concrete sense, or what it means for an entity like light to "behave as a wave and as a particle." However—going back to pragmatism and to Albers' color theory—atoms are a *useful*, "actual" model of how the world works. Wave and particle behavior are successfully predicted, and defined formally, by mathematical equations, but this does not obliterate the possibility that nonwave or nonparticle shapes or entities—however visualized or conceptualized—might eventually better explain broader dynamics of physical systems. In the meantime, we use waves and particles as acceptable geometric essentialisms for these bumbling systems. What, then, about other essentialisms, such as social categories, or the separation of "individuals" from "situations"?[25]

Emirbayer and Mische (1998) discuss "situationisms" as essentialist from the standpoint of postulating actors and situations as somehow neatly separable. Practically, there are good reasons for thinking about treating them as distinct. False dualisms of agents and their structures, such as "men and their moments" (Goffman 1967, 3), are replaced by a relational pragmatics of *transactions*—not in terms of moral responsibility for individual actions, but in terms of how dignity might be developed. Dignity is about the transactive and practical nature of social life, not about neat or sharp divides between selves.

Transactions, following Emirbayer, are situated encounters in which actors are present as constituted by each of their own previous encounters, then mutually changed throughout each new encounter and as a matter of perceiving each other and each other's actions. If we stay the same, in terms of having a personality or consistency of behavior, this is a product of consistent environments and consistent people within those environments (see also Alwin, Cohen, and Newcomb 1991). The focus here is on external influences, not a putative internal consistency.

Emirbayer (1997) classifies norm-driven and material-economic approaches to individual action as essentialist, in the sense of viewing social

---

[25] John Levi Martin (2003) details a version of this logic in explicating field theory, ultimately ending up in approximately the opposite position to ours in terms of the utility of thinking of internal processes as important for understanding social action. In this book, we will employ the concept as an indicator of social circumstances, not a cause, but we hold open the possibility that seeking to achieve this internal sense—whatever is—does drive some social action.

interaction as a phenomenon occurring according to singular social forces, between discrete or "separate" individuals, or within or against particular socioeconomic or capital backdrops. While there is no mistaking the fact that norms can be especially useful for understanding given behaviors or lines of action (Swidler 2001), essentialisms might still tend to posit and reify social forces as if they are prescriptive. Alternatively, a relational pragmatic perspective, as we outline here in keeping with Emirbayer, not only traces individuality proper to society but also views "rational thought" as inseparable from the emotionally charged contexts and motivations. People are not isolated organisms, studied by focusing only on their individual properties. Rather, information from and about those individuals is nested within an understanding—and ideally measurement—of the wider social circles, processes, and regularities they inhabit. Much sociological research already captures these rich approaches to individuals, situations, and life chances (e.g., Frye 2012, 2019), but the question is how we might think about dignity in a way that similarly reflects this conceptual and methodological commitment to relational pragmatism.

Overall, dignity can be perceived to be at stake in ways that are both tiny and smaller and bigger or much larger, adding to an individual's overall sense of subjective dignity over time. In principle, this would be like how an individual's overall sense of mastery or control over their life (see Haidt and Rodin 1999 for one overview) reflects a combination of numerous life situations and events, some of which are privately deemed more pivotal or influential than others, ranging from dropping a frying pan in the kitchen to experiencing job loss.

Goffmanian approaches to dignity emphasize poise and avoiding embarrassment through one's actions and appearance. If one can absorb any awkwardness within interaction or draw attention away from it by using confidence or social skill, then did indignity actually occur, and if so how and for whom? The answers to these sorts of practical questions might exist within the eyes of the beholders. When stand-up comedians joke about certain wardrobe taboos such as wearing Crocs to a business interview, is dignity really at stake, or something much milder?[26] The way people experience the social gravity of an action depends on its context.

In the final analysis, while there is much individual creativity involved in how people define and redefine the situations they are in, coordination

---

[26] Thank you to Chris Pieper for this example.

of social action relies on minimally shared definitions of situations. These shared understandings of what happens at a bus stop, a concert, or a classroom are a basis of what it would mean to achieve dignity within those situations. One way of reclaiming dignity would be to redefine a situation in the moment, by sharing information or asserting a different identity to change midstream how others view oneself—or how one views oneself. Extreme forms of indignity, such as violence or abuse, are likely to transcend to situational characteristics and thus reliably threaten dignity.

## People as Ends/Reasons: Becoming Dignified by Living through and for Others

While a practical or embodied approach to dignity has the advantage of realistically expanding the definitional framework and applicability of dignity, it also risks trivializing dignity in the same stride. If morality, like dignity, is potentially endlessly dynamic, how does this advance social science? How do we keep dignity from *meaning too little* within a framework like this?

To elide the brute reality of categorization would be to ignore much of what matters to dignity. So, how can we incorporate a relational pragmatic approach without undermining the hierarchical and categorical insights so important to how we think about and enact dignity in America or within any other society marked by varying forms of social inequality? Perhaps one solution to integrating categorical and personal, relational realities resides in staying mindful of how individuals experience and relate to categories as lived realities and, of course, amid social interaction. *The experience of difference is relational before it is categorical: it depends on where we live and the company we keep* (Monk 2022).

A transactional approach to society replaces social interactions with multiple defined situations and purely autonomous people with the transactive nature of existence, refusing to posit social individuals as discrete entities and instead viewing them as engaged subjects who experience socially granted autonomy as they build selves and persons—as residues of experience accumulate and settle within each person.

Breaking the assumption of discrete individuals in the name of relational pragmatism and replacing it with a web of life not only is a statistical inconvenience for population science but also raises a basic, fundamental issue. When we participate in society, we participate as individuals and are regarded as such, and so the reality of society is one in which individual personhood is recognized and reproduced as a matter of dignity's sanctity. One question, then, becomes how personhood is experienced in ways that are more discrete and ways that are more relational, and how these viewpoints might be applied jointly—toward the ultimate benefit of a more integrated understanding of how dignity works.

How distinct we *think* we are as individuals is separate from how distinct we *actually* are, and this rehearsed, perceived chasm is a fundamentally social one, as some national cultures emphasize independence, while others tend to emphasize interdependence (Markus and Kitayama 1991; Shweder 1991). Drawing practical lines between ourselves and those with whom we interact is not so simple. Each of us participates in our own mental experience by designating some thoughts as typical of ourselves or "belonging" to us (James 1892). An absence of perceived social coercion allows us to convince ourselves that some thoughts are "authentic" to ourselves (e.g., Turner 1976).

The same is true of action: mental health accompanies the ability to convince ourselves that we steered our actions; otherwise we might feel resentful if we do not respect the marching orders, or we might begin to lose our sense of control or autonomy over our own lives, not to mention our sanity. Dignity as a social process involves this translation of external circumstances into at least the *perception* of internal freedom. It is in part a coming around to the fact that I endorse what I do and what I do represents who I am.

In other words, some essentialisms are necessary fictions for the proper operation of social life, both inside and outside the social institutions of social science. We hold individuals responsible as accountable agents, both interpersonally and legally. Functionally rational thought in society is impossible without a recognition of a self, even as the tools and material guiding the rationality are social.

The Penn State philosopher Sarah Clark Miller (2017) asks whether any pure rationality might be reconceptualized considering how care propels reason. She sees this reconceptualization as a tool for "reconsidering dignity." People significant to us inform our reasoning or even become reasons in their own right. People themselves are not rational, yet to us they become rational sources of information for why we do what we do.

Dignity highlights the impossibility of existing without being recognized. Developmental neuroscience has established that the conscious mind is formed—brought online from a hazy unintelligibility—through an internalization of the language, gestures, and habits of our caregivers. No thought has ever been solely our own, and no thought ever will be. An individual mind is a mentalization of others' presumed mental states. And yet we are autonomous in terms of how each of our minds experiences identity and organizes and deploys thoughts and actions accordingly.

Committing to particular life projects or significant others leads us, in practice, to value what those commitments imply. We do not choose our value commitments, but rather we are chosen by them over the course of our personal experience by the people with whom we transact over time: values are felt prolongations of particular social experiences and particular people into the self (Berger and Luckmann 1966; Joas 2000; see also Miles 2015). Values are self-evident responses to the world that make practical sense within individual lives, but they do not always usefully predict what we will do or say in a given situation: how we will talk or what we will do in order to defend ourselves from uncertainty, embarrassment, or shame (Goffman 1963; Mills 1959; Swidler 1986, 2001; Vaisey 2009).

We can shift the view a little if we take seriously Dan-Cohen's (2011) assertion that "morality requires first and foremost respect for others' dignity rather than for one's own" (15).[27] Sheer recognition of another person (Ricoeur 1992)—by seeing them, saying their name, or remembering them—makes an intersubjective demand upon us as a real potential for a "deliberative setting off of (individual) persons" (Debes 2009).

At the outset of any social interaction, when we look *at someone,* we *see someone,* if only to reflexively deny what we have seen, as in the case of war combat or mass genocide. One might even advance a theory of posttraumatic stress disorder among combat veterans by pointing out a socialization of lack of dignity of the enemy that is necessary to warrant and motivate killing: this dehumanization serves an instrumental purpose, but its basis in a revocation of human dignity becomes all too apparent once one has left the battlefield, leading to extreme cognitive dissonance that may never be adequately resolved to satisfaction.[28] Like Sulmasy (2007), the philosopher Stephen Darwall separates the fact of having seen someone from the choice of what to do given that recognition. Recognition of others is a prerequisite of one's own dignity. What happens next is a matter of situation and agency.

---

[27] Following Sulmasy's distinction between intrinsic and attributed dignity, what one does in response to this moral recognition, or how one interprets it cognitively or linguistically, adds another, more complicated layer, and likely varies across social groups and societies throughout history.

[28] Thank you to Professor Carson Mencken for providing this example.

In this phenomenological, real sense, dignity intrinsically represents "unearned worth," which then may be dishonored through marginalization, stigma, or other forms of structural inequality. This brute fact (Smith 2009) is "central to any reflection on the nature of human worth" (Debes 2009). Similarly, Darwall has referred to the social basis of dignity as "the irreducibly second-personal character of both our dignity and the kind of respect that is its appropriate response."

Hegel makes another point that is no less crucial: freedom and recognition are two sides of the same experiential coin, or as Giddens (1984) puts it, society constrains and enables us as individuals to an extent shaped by culture. We cannot feel free without others recognizing or upholding our freedom on a continual basis, and, vitally, we must also perceive others as free when they are relating to us for that relation to be meaningful to ourselves. Relatedly, Simmel (1950) spoke of "freedom for some purpose," essentially contending that structural latitude in individual action only is interpreted as such within and against that structure. Cultures—and individuals within them—valorize freedom toward certain ends and not others. The freedom to rearrange paper clips on one's desk or select which Netflix show to watch might be seen as less important than the freedom to work at home or resist mundane requests from tense people. Some freedoms are viewed as trivial or not worth exploiting (Emirbayer and Mische 1994).

## Reasoning Follows (Lack of) Caring about People

Consider Happy, an intelligent elephant that (or who) can recognize itself in a mirror.[29] In a recent legal case calling for Happy's release from the Bronx Zoo, philosophical questions relevant to animal rights and dignity arose, such as, "How much intelligence do you have to have to be able to be autonomous?" The University of Chicago philosopher Martha Nussbaum, who testified in the case, maintained the view that it is "bad" to predicate animal rights on a presumed likeness to human life. When it comes to speciesism, might apparently makes right, since human ethics have shaped the control and destruction of animal populations. But how rational are humans, really?

So much of our culture is informed by, or exists in reaction to, humanity's presumed rational capacity, or ability to reason or think logically and

---

[29] "The Elephant in the Courtroom," *New Yorker*, March 7, 2022.

"independently" as separate persons. Kant and others based their moral edifices on this potential. Much of the academic and professional discipline of economics posits rationality as the basis for understanding human decisions, although behavioral economics represents a tidal shift in terms of understanding the many ways that people act against their stated interests or what would in fact optimize their outcomes, thanks largely to social or contextual "biases" (Kahneman 2011; Thaler 2016; Tversky and Kahneman 1974). An ability to make decisions and evaluate oneself and others takes many forms, but a notion of people as mathematically maximizing options and opportunities is a potent, if flawed, one: one that plays into the cultural fixation on quantification and mastery of life through numbers (Lupton 2016), as Weber noted.

Individuals are not economically rational, in terms of always getting the most out of every situation they are in, however that might be defined or measured. Rather, individuals are *imaginatively rational* (Lakoff and Johnson 2008): they optimize based on how they frame or interpret situations, based on their social experiences. Individuals cogitate by drawing analogies to other or inferred experiences, not by balance sheets. These analogies and metaphors shift in interaction midstream, as individuals speak and relate, part of the creative fluidity inherent to social life. While a bit passé for us to tear down the already mortally wounded notion of man as *homo economicus*, that atomistic sense of rationality is often appealed to as the core of human dignity, the core capacity that separates us from animals, robots, and small children.

C. Wright Mills' (1940) pivotal work on vocabularies of motive positions rationality itself as rationalization—that is, grounded in the legitimacy of situational vocabularies—and metaphors as collectively interwoven with emotion and motivation (Lakoff and Johnson 2008). Notions of "thinking for oneself," "getting ahead," "being fair," "profiting," and other ways of assessing individuals and their discrete, autonomous gains are based on how individuals have seen these turns of language applied within other, seemingly analogous situations.

Even an economically brute logic like "viewing money as the real motive" is fundamentally dependent on what individuals view as a proper "payoff" and under which specific or applied circumstances. Money and its supposedly "natural" motivations are socially shaped (e.g., Zelizer 2010). In this same vein, Hegel offers a deep critique of rationality when he associates it with a conflation of natural law and capitalist superstructures: what is "rational" is relational. Rationality in any presumed "pure" form bespeaks "a purely metaphysical conception of man."

Dignity "rejects all utilitarian justification" and is a matter of "practical consensus" (Debes 2009). Further, on Debes' account, dignity "purports to allege the existence of a kind of moral community between humans." Pragmatically, we live for those whom we have known or know. Kantian thought has usefully proposed "seeing into" the lives of others. Michèle Lamont similarly locates dignity as an interpersonal, situated process of, as she says, what the philosopher Axel Honneth called recognition: "a social act by which the positive social worth of an individual or group is affirmed or acknowledged by others." To put the idea negatively, Albert Camus once said, "I was looked at, but I wasn't seen." An objectifying gaze and a look of recognition might spell a difference between dignity and its lack. Thus, we build upon relational understandings between selves to bracket dignity's supposed rational basis; the whole process is social, even its rational parts.

Issues of how and when to care—and whom to care about—constitute what we call morality, or the duties and obligations and proscriptions that people live by in a society, a polity, or a tribe. In this sense, morality is fundamentally anchored in emotional processes, as Hume famously argued in response to Kant's focus on morality's logical basis. The extent to which something *is* moral is reflected in the degree of emotional response it elicits either when enacted or when violated (Hitlin and Vaisey 2013; Luft 2020). Given how morality ultimately is a situated and local project—it takes place within one's moral community—being "good enough" often involves justifying behavior that an outsider might view as immoral (Hitlin 2008).

Not only is Kant's pure rationality made impure by the interpersonal, but also it's hopelessly interwoven with and impelled by emotion. As Wharton professor Adam Grant tweeted, "Being rational isn't about eliminating your emotions. It's about harnessing them to inform your judgment instead of letting them cloud your judgment." Here, Grant is correct, in that emotions prefigure our thinking through deep intuitions and sentiments. And while one can be "too emotional," from a cultural standpoint of emotion norms or feeling rules (Hochschild 1979; Von Scheve 2012; Wingfield 2010), or in ways that make rationalistic[30] thinking difficult, emotion always infuses judgment. What is social is moral and vice versa.

---

[30] Thinking that seems "rational" or "reasonable" to oneself or when verbalized to those who participate within a given social context.

In this sense, Grant usefully echoes Adam Smith's theory of moral sentiments. Rationality and emotionality represent a unity, not a duality. They are mutually constitutive rather than diametrically opposed. Dignity is emotionally driven around dispositions, beliefs, and practices and correspondingly hard to define apart from them as they are experienced.

And yet, though perhaps as expected in a bureaucratic age of rationalization and standardization, a mystique of dignity through calculation still holds allure. Modern economic and scientific triumphs have generally upheld an apotheosis of calculation and evidence-based practice, with many societal benefits resulting in terms of social efficiency and individual legal or bodily protection (Espeland and Sauder 2007; Gauchat 2015). Ironically, though, Smith's own work is used to promote reason as the source of humanity's salvation despite the corpus of his thought, which, in totality, sees the important role of human sympathy for optimizing—and reining in—markets or efficiencies. Structures do not know how to use themselves: only individuals within structures can come to that determination. It seems that, after all these centuries, we still are fixated on the socially defined logical abilities of our minds—they can solve equations—and less on the fact that logic, in most senses outside of pure mathematics, is profoundly emotional, moral, or care based.

When Kant described the human person as "the subject of a morally practical reason," he nodded to the practical nature of morality. For Schopenhauer, concepts and emotions derive their human value from each other, not apart from each other. In the traditions of Hume and Rousseau, perception and compassion are prior to rationality and shape it in ways that prefigure the scope of thinking that takes place. Modern neuroscience has vindicated many of these philosophical insights.

Modern neuroscience (e.g., Damasio 1994, 1999; Phelps and LeDoux 2005) demonstrates that even rational decision-making relies on a core emotional substrate. When emotional substrates of the brain, such as the amygdala, are damaged, people struggle to make basic decisions. What feels right to us *is* right for us: we depend on feeling to reason, rather than the other way around. When students take exams in chemistry or math, they are recalling and applying facts in a quintessentially rational manner, but the social world, as a moral realm, does not have an answer key or set of formally rendered rules. Rather, the social world carries a set of legitimate values and commitments toward which individuals change their relations and intuitions over time, as a practical matter.

As Hodgkiss points out, Kant, Kierkegaard, and Nietzsche all paint emotionality in a negative light, a kind of weakness in the hard dealings of life. Many philosophers have apparently experienced a vested interest in their promotion of rationality-as-salvation, assuming that with an overemphasis on emotion or compassion—which are conflated with "irrationality"—civilization will collapse. This dismissal of compassion bespeaks a larger intellectual trend in many corners of Continental philosophy: a reigning Cartesian dualism that imagines the mind as having its own cool, paneled chamber where it calculates at a padded desk and is unmoved by life's animations.

Indeed, the phenomenologist Maurice Merleau-Ponty, whose work informs modern pragmatist thought, conceived of knowledge as "felt": "Our bodies think and know in ways that precede cognition."[31] The interdisciplinary field of social neuroscience has since developed and tested models to elucidate this. Jonathan Haidt's (2001) social intuitionist model draws on neuroscience and psychology research to position rational thought as a "rider" astride the "elephant" of the subconscious, emotional mind and its bodily substrates. Similarly, a dual-process model, widely accepted across the social sciences, positions thinking as a post hoc set of rationalist or socially legitimated vocabularies for justifying what we truly care about or have done—which are our commitments or deeply vested interests.[32] Rationality and emotionality are interwound subconsciously, regardless of how much we might talk about their clean separation. Being "level-headed" is a matter of emotional intelligence. Hume, for example, always construed reason at the intersection of reason and sentiment, famously positing rationality to be slave to the passions.[33]

Our stated values for stimulation, achievement, self-direction, benevolence, power, hedonism, or conformity, for example, can be measured (Hitlin and Piliavin 2004; Schwartz and Bilsky 1987; Schwartz 2017), but they are experienced as bigger than oneself, important guides toward which we orient our actions and our senses of self (Hitlin 2008). The fact they do a relatively poor job of predicting individual behavior in specific situations, since situations have unique demands, speaks to how our stated values take shape depending on what others want and how we relate to others.[34]

---

[31] Quoted in *Landmarks* by Robert Macfarlane (1996).

[32] This is but only a passing point for us, and the field has a lot to say about whether there are really two processes, and how and when they are intertwined. We elide all of that for our purposes, that people have thoughts and feelings that are complicatedly intertwined; our basic point is that they are socially shaped and channeled and underlie our subsequent theory of dignity-in-society.

[33] Haidt (2006) makes this a central theme in his work on healthy psychological functioning.

[34] See Martin and Lembo (2020) for a very skeptical take on the concept of values in social science.

Personal identity, "a sense of self built up over time as the person embarks on and pursues projects or goals" (Hewitt 1997, 93), is a source of "achieved coherence" (Hitlin 2003). Values are only one source of identity, becoming personal as they are enacted.

## Conclusion

Recent re-engagement with morality in the social sciences (e.g., Abend 2008; Bargheer 2018; Gray and Graham 2018; Haidt 2001; Hitlin and Vaisey 2013) suggests a more realistic approach to how individuality looks and feels, moving beyond some rational calculating machine or a jumble of emotions. In any society, moral convictions are experienced as emotional and they form a core of deliberative judgment across varying interpersonal or relational contexts (Hitlin 2008; Smith 2003; Taylor 1991).

Morality and dignity are local, operating within social relationships and through acts of caring or neglect. The basis for a moral self has been shifting toward a more self-directed notion of what is "true" or good for an individual who now has the right to pursue her own interests, sometimes at a cost to groups or institutions (Bellah et al. 1985; Turner 1987), part of a modernization process that traces back at least to Tocqueville's analysis.[35] Nobody is a priori better than anybody else, captured in notions of universal human rights that have seen transnational momentum among democratic governments (Habermas 2010).

In parallel, Taylor (1991) suggests a shift from what was once anchoring our sense of morality in God or The Good toward the "massive subjective turn of modern culture" (26). People soon discover their place within social webs of understanding, participating in what Heinz (2002) called "self-socialization." The tools that our societies, groups, friends, and workplaces give us for evaluating actions—our own and others'—enmesh us in moralities that we use to anchor our own senses of self, as moral (enough) beings (Hitlin 2008).

However individualistic our society might seem, morality has been, and always will be, *personal*—precisely because it is *interpersonal*. Dignity reflects an interaction between morality and emergent individuality, and that

---

[35] See Kashima, Foddy, and Platow (2002) for one brief overview.

interaction is mediated by experiences of caring for others. This leaves the content of experienced dignity up to the interpretations of a person being asked. However, the personal intertwining of one's feelings of worthiness in the eyes of others offers us leverage on the relationship between people and the social structures they live within.

# 4

# American Capitalism and Its
# Multifaceted Links to Dignity

In this chapter, we focus on American capitalism as a superstructure, or interwoven set of social structures, that shapes individual dignity through resource- and stress-based mechanisms before and during the Covid-19 pandemic. Building on the last chapter's insights, we only learn who we are by interacting with others within wider social structures that predate us, and in America, those structures are infused with cultural and legal understandings of capitalism. These structures, in turn, shape the social conditions through which we achieve dignity in a capitalist society.

Whether through one's labor or one's ownership of property, capitalism involuntarily marries individuals to social quantifications of their worth, even as individuals experience themselves as priceless. This specifically occurs through multiple, interlinked forms of structured inequality (Figure 4.1).

Building on the insights of earlier chapters, we know that historical conditions of particular social groups are linked to expectations and biases related to these groups, which in turn have the potential to impact group-specific dignity levels. For instance, as we see in Figure 4.1, groups defined by social class, race, sex, ability, or age have differing average positions within a capitalist system. *Capitalism favors social groups that possess capital, often not by explicit policy but rather by privileging availability of money, time, or energy, all of which feed into what we call "opportunity."* Hence, classism, racism, sexism, and ableism all are built into capitalism. Worker dignity within capitalism is shaped both inside and outside of the workplace, by one's affordances for autonomy, flexibility, and skill utilization on the job, and by the resources one has for pursuing a desired life while not on the clock.

As we begin to map out here, one's perceived dignity exists within or against economic relations. Tension between observer and personal accounts of dignity is to be expected. An observer looking through

*The Science of Dignity.* Steven Hitlin and Matthew A. Andersson, Oxford University Press.
© Oxford University Press 2023. DOI: 10.1093/oso/9780197743867.003.0005

| | | | | |
|---|---|---|---|---|
| | → | Classism | | Distribution |
| Historical & Social | → | Racism | → | of |
| Conditions of Capitalism | → | Sexism | ← | Dignity |
| | → | Ableism | | in America |

**Figure 4.1**  Linking Capitalism to Structural Biases (-Isms) That Influence Dignity in America

capitalism's shop window might dispute a worker's account of their so-called dignity. Still, an individual's belief in their own dignity is bound to have real consequences.

## Dignity in American Capitalism: How Do Individuals and Inequalities Connect?

In Chapter 2, we distinguished between average- and variation-based ways of viewing population health. We are all "in this together"; we are "free and equal"; all lives are invaluable—and yet we live unequal existences with differing life expectancies attached to them (Geronimus et al. 2019; Montez et al. 2021). As economists point out, plenty of other high-income nations underwent industrial, economic, labor, and educational expansions like the United States over the past century and yet contained social and health inequalities within narrower ranges (Montez et al. 2019; Reynolds 2021). Elizabeth Popp Berman (2022) charts tradeoffs between efficiency and equity in America: as it turns out, even Democrats are reined in by a fear of overspending that impedes their social ambitions.

Max Weber (1981, 139) pointed to "disenchantment" (*Entzauberung*) as one of the more serious injuries of modernity, itself a kind of religion: "that one can, in principle, master all things by calculation." Capitalism is nothing if not numbers oriented. We are by turns excited and numbed by numbers. Profits, overhead, talent, and rankings all are valorized quantities (Espeland and Sauder 2007). The very capacity of numbers to seem "true" and objective—even independently of their applications—contributes to their usage as a core aspect of modern rationality.

Numbers cannot tell us how they should be used, but they are tools that have gained legitimacy as rationalism has: a self-evident sort of social legitimacy, numbers for numbers' sake, "capable of establishing their own axiomatics (through the fundamental tautology 'business is business,' on which 'the economy' is based)" (Bourdieu 1990, 113).

Capitalism takes different forms in different countries.[1] For instance, Nordic countries are generous with work flexibility and paid leave in ways that trickle down to better child health,[2] and France forbids workers to eat lunch at their desks.[3] Still, much is the same in the United States and elsewhere: capitalism involves economic and social structures premised on returns on capital. Capital assumes diverse forms with ultimate reference to money (Bourdieu 1986), such as property, wealth, skill, acculturation, or networks. Human capital, in the form of skilled labor, is counted up and counted on to convert economic and material investments continually and efficiently into socially valued outputs that are priced and sold in diverse markets.

Conversions among financial, human, material, social, and cultural capitals seem quintessential to understanding not only capitalism's dynamics (Bourdieu 1986) but also the (un)dignified involvement of individuals within living these dynamics. When millions feel like they cannot get ahead no matter how hard they work, this speaks not only to positional advantages in society but also to the different rates of return attached to different forms of capital. Due to differences in their social, economic, or occupational positions, different individuals command different returns on their efforts, with individuals who possess more capital generally occupying higher positions and generating higher economic returns across time. This can be captured in many ways, for instance, by focusing on cumulative inequality in wealth, income, or other economic advantages.

### Indignity across the American Class Structure: Hard Realities and Looking the Other Way

Working conditions hardly are similar across "good jobs," which are salaried and professional, and "bad jobs," which are wage based and precarious (Kalleberg 2009, 2018), and yet these jobs all are profoundly shaped by an economy that emphasizes routinization, standardization, automation,

---

[1] As documented, for example, in Gøsta Esping-Andersen's (1990) *Three Worlds of Welfare Capitalism*.

[2] Andersson, Garcia, and Glass (2021).

[3] "Drop That Fork! Why Eating at Your Desk Is Banned in France," National Public Radio, June 10, 2022.

output, and metrics of performance. Recently, the cultural essayist Eula Biss (2020, 149) quoted Studs Terkel's *Working*: "The blue-collar blues is no more bitterly sung than the white-collar moan." Further, Biss observed: "Blue collar and white call upon the identical phrase: 'I'm a robot.'" While some working conditions are far more physically hazardous or riskier relative to others, few jobs are uniformly easy, and many of us fear becoming cogs in an organizational machine whose dynamics remain mysterious.

In a recent issue of the *British Journal of Sociology*, Lamont (2019, 660) maintains that an American dream based in wealth accumulation through hard work is losing collective appeal as fewer people are, or feel like they are, getting ahead based on their skills or effort. She observes a shared crisis across the social class spectrum, but with distinct reasons at the top compared to the bottom: the upper-middle class, she writes, is afflicted by an "intensified diffusion of neoliberal scripts of the self" (see also Hall and Lamont 2013) involving the working, toiling rich. Similarly, the middle and upper-middle classes face pressures to work, deliver, innovate, and perform. As Erin Cech (2021) shows, overwork continues to perpetuate under the guise of self-fulfillment: "following your passion" presumes a level of economic safety that few actually achieve, and it leads to tremendous personal sacrifice. Meanwhile, lower-income and working-class individuals are being disproportionately shut out from stable livelihoods—they "do not have the resources needed to live the dream."

This collective diagnosis across the social class spectrum—one of "shared disillusionment, differing class-based maladies," in Lamont's words— mirrors the conclusions of the political philosopher Michael Sandel in *Tyranny of Merit*: that is, general distress and constrained opportunities for dignification both at the top and at the bottom of the occupational and economic hierarchies, with differing reasons for disillusionment across the hierarchy. Even more, Lamont writes, racial and ethnic groups confronted with historical and cultural discrimination "face (even) more rigid boundaries" keeping them from success or social worth.

Sennett and Cobb ([1972] 1993) spoke in *Hidden Injuries of Class* about how America's class structure "is organized so that the tools of freedom [such as education] become sources of indignity" (30). Moreover, they observed that this structure is upheld if not extolled by the alienating myth that mechanically ascending the ranks will lead to "more development of internal powers" (58). Lamont (2000) observed these cross-class indignities firsthand. Middle- and upper-middle-class dignification is caught up in the intense work and postural pressures of large-scale, corporatized bureaucracies, while working-class dignity involves hard work that contrasts itself against the "insincerity" of white-collar jobs that involve manipulation—a styled manipulation of data, needs, or inputs—rather than "honest" manual labor. Andrew Sayer made a similar point when he stated that occupational rank or dominance might be easily confused with dignity, but they are hardly the same thing (2007, 2011). Even under conditions of "participative management," workplace relations in modern bureaucratic environments seem unable to get back to what they once were preindustrially, what Hodson (1996, 719) calls an "incomplete recovery of the positive experiences of craft production."

What social philosophers and social scientists alike are coming to recognize is the "invisible complexity" (Bellah et al. 1985) connecting workers across the entire economy to their organizational and postindustrial fates. Even as we work among actual people, "iron cages"[4] hold us captive, numbing our subjective wills. Likewise, an immense technocracy connects political and economic institutions to the public will (Sandel 2020).

## Myths of Mobility

Social mobility in America is declining and incomes for most workers are stagnant. Judging by the number of work hours alone, there is no straightforward association between income and time spent working, or between social mobility and time spent working. Instead, based on decades of confidential tax return data analyzed for the Equality of Opportunity project based at Stanford University, income and social mobility are far more correlated with family background and educational credentials.[5]

In an economy where getting ahead is as much (if not more) about one's family and educational origins as it is about present toil, what can be said for worker dignity? One need not look beyond an Amazon warehouse, nursing home, or fast-food restaurant to quickly get a sense of how humans can be worked to the brink of sheer exhaustion. Likewise, one need not look beyond

---

[4] Max Weber, *The Protestant Ethic and the Spirit of Capitalism*, translated by Talcott Parsons. New York: Scribner, 1958.

[5] For our purposes, we are eliding a related discussion about the American belief that this is a meritocracy. This belief is powerful; the evidence suggests we are far from a society where everyone has an equal chance to succeed. This is a key issue, but tangential to our focus.

hospitals or law firms to get a sense of how some highly paid professionals are losing sleep.

Recent political and economic developments, such as labor market segmentation by college education and the intensification of nonlabor capital returns over labor income returns, have decoupled a once-strong relationship between hard work and getting by, not to mention wealth accumulation. Inequality-generating processes in America today are seen as mysterious by many, or even overlooked entirely, even as we hold fast to commonly held values of work, success, and family.

Hard work nowadays often is associated with hourly wage work that involves scheduling instability, or even second or third shifts at other jobs (Kalleberg 2009, 2018; Schneider and Harknett 2019). Meanwhile, higher-earning workers hardly are immune from overwork. The "stress of higher status" (e.g., Schieman and Koltai 2017) comes with overtime at the medical clinic or the legal or financial firm. There is no business without busyness, or so Oliver Burkeman observes in a recent *Wall Street Journal* editorial on the efficiency trap: "The more productive we are, the more pressure we feel."[6] Meanwhile, many Americans' lack of access to job quality and safety figures prominently, as noted by recent American Sociological Association president Christine Williams (2021).

In recent decades, adults in America have come to view financial stability or success as one of the more common ways to a satisfying life, and a rewarding career generally ranks among the top perceived ways to life satisfaction or happiness (Pew Research Center 2021). Moreover, with committed relationships and having children also remaining prized life goals, we face profound internal conflicts as workers and as humans, when much of society experiences work and family as competing (e.g., Blair-Loy 2003).

Lamont contrasts the *individual* resilience that our economy prizes—the grittiness and consistency of a humanoid—with the *social* resilience afforded by policies and laws that make people belong or feel like they matter or are understood (Hall and Lamont 2013). Yet, American society has somehow become structurally complicit in opposing these humanitarian values. Most individuals would prefer less economic inequality than they believe exists (Pew Research Center 2020), and the level of inequality they believe exists generally is far less than actually exists. The America we want is not the

---

[6] Oliver Burkeman, "Escaping the Efficiency Trap—and Finding Some Peace of Mind," Wall Street Journal, August 6, 2021.

America we have, and valuing hard work and wealth at the same time as fairness or social justice leads to great internal conflict as to how to resolve our economic predicament.

We seem to be collectively looking the other way. Americans egregiously overestimate rates of social mobility, underestimate income inequality, underestimate wealth inequality, underestimate the ratio of CEO to worker pay, and underestimate racial wealth inequality, regardless of whether they come from advantaged or disadvantaged social backgrounds (Kiatpongsan and Norton 2014; Kraus et al. 2019; Norton and Ariely 2011). A 2015 article in *Scientific American*[7] explains that part of the reason for such collective ignorance of the economic facts lies in persistent optimism: specifically, optimism attached to hard work, part of the American Dream. Not unrelatedly, inequality is perceived to be fair or deserved, due to how Americans connect hard work to merit (Mijs 2021; Starmans, Sheskin, and Bloom 2017).

Perhaps the facts would deal too strong a blow to our motivation or investment in the status quo. This inverse link between ideal-worker ideology and actively searching for new facts about social inequality suffuses American thinking. In fact, a belief in hard work *is* higher in societies *with* higher amounts of income inequality, speaking to how citizens literally come to justify inequality through the hard work that supposedly generates it. This holds even when all segments of the population are working hard, and even when inequalities in work hours are not nearly on the same scale as income and wealth inequality (Mijs 2021). Money and morality are allied (Zelizer 1979, 1994): what is economically rich is deemed—from the standpoint of how inequality is understood—morally and politically right.

Individuals are most motivated to learn more about what they already believe, a ubiquitous process termed "confirmation bias." Thus, Marx might suggest America as an exemplar of what he termed "a state of false consciousness," which involves citing presumed personal shortcomings as the reasons for why we think we remain relatively poor, precarious, or unwealthy. Part of this so-called ignorance might be completely practical: regardless of what we believe, we still need to wake up and go to work tomorrow. The world is a bit more comforting if it seems like we have earned our successes and others have earned their relative lack of success.

Rates of poverty and financial hardship remain unusually high in the United States, where poverty is durable and distressing given a lack of social

---

[7] Nicholas Fitz, "Economic Inequality: It's Far Worse Than You Think," March 31, 2015.

resources and high costs of living (Grusky and Hill 2018). Meanwhile, some media commentators with tens of millions of viewers miss the point of American poverty's generally unlivable and overwhelming nature by instead fixating on exceptional cases of upward social mobility—"rags to riches" or viral influencers—or on how America's poorest technically belong in the global middle class.

Part of the picture of American poverty stems from what could have been. Counterfactual income analyses show that incomes below the 90th percentile should be 30% to 70% higher than they are today, based on how economic productivity mapped onto average worker pay up until the 1970s.[8] The historically widening gap between American economic success and average worker compensation has come to be by increased income and wealth inequality between elites and average workers, beginning around the 1970s.

Income and wealth inequality have reached historic highs (Grusky and Hill 2018),[9] prompting many to locate the emergence of ultra-wealthy and billionaire social classes. While inequality alone is not an explanation for poverty (McCall 2013), rising inequality in itself does not significantly trickle down to less poverty, and a privatization of wealth leaves fewer options for addressing poverty as a social problem. In societies where income inequality is high, social mobility is indeed lower, with primary and secondary educational systems linked to community tax bases serving as channeling mechanisms, linking the geographic segregation of family wealth to the adult earnings and occupational placements of the next generation (Bloome, Dyer, and Zhou 2018; Jerrim and Macmillan 2015; Reardon 2011).

## American Inequities before and during the Covid-19 Pandemic

A lack of systematic attention to worker well-being and security is odd given American circumstances. Increased national economic activity generally correlates with tolerance, self-direction, and civic or public engagement

---

[8] "America's 1% Has Taken $50 Trillion from the Bottom 90%," *TIME* magazine, September 14, 2020; "Trends in Income from 1975 to 2018" and "A $2.5 Trillion Question: What If Incomes Grew Like GDP Did?," Working Papers, RAND Corporation, 2020.

[9] In addition to sources in the previous footnote, see also, e.g., "Piketty's Inequality Story in Six Charts," *New Yorker,* March 2014; "How Political Ideas Keep Economic Inequality Going," *Harvard Gazette,* March 2020; and "A Guide to Statistics on Historical Trends in Income Inequality," Center on Budget and Policy Priorities, January 2020.

(Inkeles 1969; Schnittker 2013). Similarly, Inglehart and Welzel (2005) demonstrate how, with national affluence, the concerns of society broaden away from a focus on preservation toward the development of specific rights and capacities for all. According to the general pattern, America's wealth should translate into wider expansion of governmental and social support, but in point of fact, we are much less equal and much less healthy than the statistics suggest we should be.

Tolls of the pandemic have spread differently by class, race, sex, physical ability, and age, deepening existing social fault lines. As sociologists have shown, "-isms" (including capitalism) operate at two key levels: structural and individual (Garcia et al. 2021; Homan 2019; Ridgeway 2011), mirroring macro and micro aspects of dignity. Structurally, "-isms" are institutionalized in terms of resources, norms, rules, or procedures that exist independently of individual people. Meanwhile, at the individual level, "-isms" manifest as personal behaviors, habits, beliefs, or preferences reflecting one's socialization, social positioning, and experience.

The -ism running throughout the others, including capitalism, is individualism: if you fail, it's on you; if you succeed, it's on you. The indignity of subscribing to a mythos of limitless freedom linked to individualism is a key reason Marx despised the term "dignity." He thought it would lift attention away from impinging structures shaping individual lives: that is, from the structural and material realities of capitalism and its fixation on numbers that numb us to the actual indignities brought about for so many by this economic system. Individualism has the benefit of fostering autonomy, one route toward mental health, but it also steals attention away from structure and thus allows many forms of structural biases to flourish.

## Classism before and during the Pandemic: The Social Chasm of a Four-Year College Degree

In a December 1, 2020, address, President Biden noted "the structural inequities in our economy that this pandemic has laid bare" and, in doing so, referred to a bifurcation of fates: those who are faring relatively well and those who have been experiencing serious economic hardships.[10] Graduating from

---

[10] Karen Ho, "US Millennials Were Grappling with the Inequality of a K-Shaped Economy Long before Covid-19," *Quartz*, December 7, 2020.

college is, to a large extent, a measurable dividing line between contrasting economic fates.

As we will cover in the analyses later, rates of food insecurity and difficulty paying bills are quite unequal by education, gender, race, and sexual orientation, among other social risk factors present during the pandemic. These stressors, in turn, are linked to the subjective dignity levels that we track. In this way, we can build on longstanding research into the college-health divide (Case and Deaton 2020; Lamont 2019; Lawrence 2017; Mirowsky and Ross 2003, 2005), feminization of poverty (McLanahan and Kelly 2006), racial inequality (Massey, Rothwell, and Domina 2009; Wilson 2012), and the elevated risk of being poor or unhoused among sexual and gender minorities (Commonwealth Fund 2021; Hsieh and shuster 2021), for example.

Congresswoman Alexandria Ocasio Cortez stated that, on principle, "there is nothing wrong with being a working person in the United States of America and there is everything dignified about it." However, the evidence unequivocally shows that higher-paying jobs among college graduates tend to be rewarding, interesting, autonomous, and satisfying relative to those not requiring a four-year college degree (Hout 2012; Mirowsky 2011; Mirowsky and Ross 2005). Indeed, the amount of flexibility, respect, and earnings that professional workers attract in America as compared to the working class is quite distinct. A lot of this has to do with the college degree divide in the labor market, and these different tracks emerge early in the hiring process. Wendy's might offer a free breakfast sandwich to its job applicants,[11] while some white-collar interviews involve paid travel and multiple paid meals.

As the Princeton economists Anne Case and Angus Deaton (2021) noted, and as sociologists have long echoed, the college divide within America is stark. Health-wise, this divide manifests as significant and considerable differences in early death and chronic disease, marked by addiction or bodily pain, by whether one obtains a four-year college degree (Lawrence 2017; Masters, Link, and Phelan 2015; Zajacova and Lawrence 2021).[12] The college divide in physical pain is significant (Zajacova et al. 2020; Zajacova, Grol-Prokopczyk, and Zimmer 2021), as is the responsibility many people place on the victims and, likewise, the divide in moral judgment between

---

[11] "Free Breakfast Sandwich with Job Application," Wendy's Coupon, Copyright 2021 Quality Is Our Recipe, LLC. Valid Only During Breakfast Hours at Wendy's. Expires 6/30/21.

[12] Associate degrees provide health and income advantages relative to no college education (Zajacova and Lawrence 2018), and possessing some college education without a two- or four-year degree can leave individuals in debt without a job and with health trajectories closer to those of high school graduates than college graduates (Zajacova and Lawrence 2021).

opioid manufacturers and those dying from addiction.[13] Economically, the college divide is present as segmentation of the labor market into "bad jobs" and "good jobs" (Kalleberg 2009, 2018). Good jobs are salaried, emphasize skillful work or autonomy, and come with more security and more benefits.[14] Precarious labor at bad jobs involves relatively low hourly wages, physically strenuous labor, little or no job security, and few worker benefits.

The differential conditions of work only widen from there. Among those without a college degree, hourly work is far more typical. As Schneider and Harknett (2019) recently found in an analysis of online survey data from retail workers across almost a hundred different big-box employers, work schedule instability—involving fluctuation in weekly hours, just-on-time scheduling practices, or "clopening," for example—is linked to psychological distress, less sleep, and general unhappiness, through pathways of work-family conflict and household financial insecurity. Most Americans have less than one thousand dollars saved to cushion any financial surprises, and consumer debt remains at an all-time high. This only adds to the elevated stress levels among those who work hourly in the service sector, wondering whether the other financial shoe will drop. Schedule instability also is related to mistrust of social institutions (Lambert, Henly, and Kim 2019). Responsibility for burnout rests on corporate cultures and employers far more than employees,[15] though in our therapeutically oriented society, it is often considered an individual's responsibility.[16] A distinct downside of a culture of individualism is existential myopia: a relative inability to see or appreciate the larger patterns shaping one's less-than-ideal circumstances.

This ratcheting up of educational bifurcation within the labor market feeds clearly into an "-ism": classism. College admissions function as an institutionalized form of classism, in at least two respects. First, as economists and sociologists of education have shown, academic ability really is an embodied mixture of cognitive or "hard" and noncognitive or "soft" skills, and these skills in turn are related to cultural capital, or socially proper familiarity with,

---

[13] An email sent between executives at AmerisourceBergen during a federal opioid trial refers to individuals living with opioid addiction as "pillbillies."

[14] Of course, these are two broad types that are not without hard-to-file examples. For instance, emergency room nurses, especially during the Covid pandemic, worked long, strenuous, and unpredictable hours while subjecting themselves to virus exposure and earning pay well above average. The point is not that all jobs fit neatly into these two types, but rather that a college education—and sometimes a two-year vocational degree—often files individuals into one or the other type.

[15] "Only Your Boss Can Cure Your Burnout," The Atlantic, March 12, 2021.

[16] Even the American Medical Association released a recommended suite of strategies for physician self-care.

attitudes toward, or expressions of intellectual ideas or topics. Being able to play the "game" of school, often with unarticulated skills and the ability to navigate certain kinds of institutions (Calarco 2014, 2018; Lareau 2011), can be inculcated in children early and serves to reproduce social classes based on a fit between structured expectations and the skills, outlooks, and attitudes that fit best into those systems (Guhin, Calarco, and Miller-Idriss 2021).

Modern economic systems produce hardships and stresses for everyone to endure; those toward the bottom of the hierarchy require more endurance and have fewer material resources or alternatives for coping. This is not conjecture: it is made abundantly clear by their greater rates of depression, illness, suicide, alcohol use, major disease, and premature death (Marmot 2015). Population research finds that the stress of higher status—overwork and work-nonwork interference being among the key indicators—pales in comparison to poverty and unstable or unrewarding work in terms of overall health effects (Schieman and Koltai 2017).

At the same time, while white-collar workers enjoy ample health and income advantages, they are hardly immune from "an environment of institutional harassment," to quote a recent Harvard Business School case at France Telecom, or one of gender discrimination, overwork, or work-family conflict, as witnessed from Silicon Valley to Wall Street and as encapsulated by glass ceilings, glass cliffs, routine overtime, and women "opting out" of the labor force at greater rates (England 2010; Goldin 2014). Meanwhile, as overviewed recently by the *Harvard Business Review*, speaking up against workplace mistreatment potentially carries its own, separate set of interpersonal and work-related risks. The presence of whistleblowers not only seems to signify healthy companies but also keeps them thriving, in terms of fewer lawsuits, lower expenses, and greater employee satisfaction.[17]

## Society's "Ideal Worker": How the Grindstone Contributes to Ableism, Sexism, Racism, and Ageism

The World Health Organization recently found that working fifty-five or more hours per week is linked to a 35% increase in the risk of stroke.[18]

---

[17] Kyle Welch and Stephen Stubben, "Throw Out Your Assumptions about Whistleblowing," *Harvard Business Review*, January 14, 2020; "Research: Whistleblowers Are a Sign of Healthy Companies," *Harvard Business Review*, November 14, 2018.

[18] "Long Working Hours Increasing Deaths from Heart Disease and Stroke," Joint News Release, World Health Organization and International Labor Organization, May 17, 2021.

Compulsive working has become its own slow-moving form of social trauma. Work both liberates us and imprisons us. Surveys tracking weekly work hours over recent decades have consistently found that Americans are working more each week, on either side of the college divide. Reasons for putting in long hours differ by occupation or job, but the fact remains that Americans are working harder than ever.

When sociologists first started noting this trend of longer hours across America about a couple decades ago, they viewed it as entangled in two mutually reinforcing developments: the intensification of work and the development of an "ideal worker" norm. The so-called ideal worker is a potent cultural myth that shapes how workers think about themselves and their performance, with some potentially brutal outcomes. An ideal worker is always available and shows a selfless devotion to their work (Blair-Loy 2003).

An ideal-worker culture transforms work into an endurance sport and workers into insecure athletes, concerned about being benched or cut with every performance. A straightforward consequence of the ideal-worker mentality is, almost by definition, an emphasis on what workers do or produce as capturing their inherent value. While some might view this as "just" the ordinary operation of market valuation, a nearsighted focus on results and exertion leads some workers to be fired or set aside and some to rise over others on account of their bodily health and fewer family obligations rather than strictly relevant ability, skill, or talent. Americans stand out for their especially taxing work hours.

Individuals who live with mental or physical disability negotiate a more restricted range of social or environmental conditions under which they can work comfortably or productively. While several larger firms have successfully integrated accommodations for individuals with disabilities, these firms typically employ college graduates and highly skilled workers, entwining classism and ableism at the organizational level. Otherwise, many small and midsized firms are ineffective or inconsistent in how they embed accommodations, leading to inequalities in retention and job satisfaction by disability status. Because age is one of the strongest predictors of disability, the effects of ageism in society are worsened by human biology: ableism and ageism are related through organic processes of diminished mental or physical capability. We return to ageism later, by relating it to negative aging stereotypes.

Ableism also influences racism in at least two important ways. First, given racial and ethnic inequalities in mental and physical health and social availability induced by multifaceted structural inequalities, whites generally have a larger stock of health and fewer social obligations as they navigate the weekly, arduous trials of being "all in" at work. Meanwhile, resulting racial and ethnic inequalities in job performance reinforce white advantages in remaining better paid in the long term and remaining employed. Being without work is itself a major risk factor for health issues through lack of financial and social resources and the stigmatization of joblessness induced by an ideal-worker culture. Further, ideal-worker cultures accelerate the process of sorting and recruiting workers in ways that team members believe, often subconsciously, are likely to result in gains or results, thus emboldening statistical discrimination.

An ideal-worker culture perpetuates sexism in other ways. Consider an unlikely yet common example: the dual-earner, heterosexual couple with kids at home. Within such couples, when the husband and wife both lead professional careers, marital or parental strain can mount over time, something exacerbated during a pandemic when parents and children are all forced to work and live in limited space. Parents show a desire to devote themselves to the successful raising of their children and inevitably they fall short on time or energy due to intense career demands around deadlines, projects, clients, traveling, or other common stressful variables in highly paid careers. While perhaps not an issue when occasional, frequent episodes of such marital or parenting stress can lead to tough conversations about what should be done to improve the climate at home.

The sociologist Youngjoo Cha (2009) has shown using longitudinal, national data that, within such dual-earner couples, a husband's long working hours is a significant trigger for the wife's quitting work, but not vice versa. In other words, even among highly educated couples, career strain linked to being an ideal worker leads to a reproduction of the traditional "separate spheres" arrangement, in which the husband works for a primary household income while the wife puts her career "on hold" to devote herself to child-rearing. This gender dynamic holds even once adjusting statistically for the incomes and career circumstances of the husband and the wife.[19] Similarly, inequalities in housework persist even among educated couples who state that they advocate gender equality.[20]

---

[19] Given current rates of college completion by gender, these powerful norms may start eroding over the next few decades, but the fact that they have not budged a great deal so far points to their obdurate nature.

[20] Claire Cain Miller, "Young Men Embrace Gender Equality, but They Still Don't Vacuum," *New York Times*, February 11, 2020.

From the standpoint of worker dignity, the sexism induced by the pressures of an ideal-worker culture leads to an important insight: worker dignity is as much about the opportunity to work as it is about what happens at work. That is, separate-spheres sexism is likely to make women feel left out of a meaningful career more so than men, when childrearing is held in the balance. This gender inequality among working parents is further cemented by the fact that "opting out" usually happens during the prime career years when promotions and raises are made or broken, making re-entries into the labor force both turbulent and unlikely to lead to the same level of success or job meaningfulness as before quitting (Goldin 2014).

A detailed window into separate spheres in the context of spousal unemployment is provided by Hayagreeva Rao's (2021) ethnographic research. Here again, double standards pertain, as a husband's unemployment is viewed as more of an urgent problem, even net of their income.

State-level paid parental leave in the United States could help to ameliorate the situation, but sexism reveals itself across years and decades, not months. Once one considers that women are *more* likely than men to earn a bachelor's degree, the fact that they are *more*, not less, likely to opt out than men puts this sexism into sharper relief. Childcare and informal elder caregiving only add to the burdens of gender inequality (England 2010; Sayer, Freedman, and Bianchi 2016). Framing caregiving as a "labor of love" tends to obscure the hard and sometimes demoralizing work that goes into it and the opportunity costs involved in terms of career or personal advancement and how these contribute to larger patterns of gender inequality.

As Hillary Clinton retweeted, "Other countries have social safety nets. The U.S. has women," referencing the sociologist Jessica Calarco's piece drawing on pre- and during-Covid scientific data on American time use.[21] As the Berkeley psychologist Alison Gopnik recently stated in a piece for *The Economist*, "Care has relied on an unstable amalgam of institutions that bridge the family, market and state. Society has depended on individual mothers and daughters, and perpetually struggling private day-care centres and nursing homes."[22] She goes on to note how the pandemic splintered this fragile arrangement, referencing how society has dangerously overworked those who provide care and left many to die alone. This all traces back, she contends, to how informal care is devalued relative to "labor" or occupational

---

[21] Jessica Calarco, "The US Social Safety Net Has Been Ripped to Shreds—and Women Are Paying the Price," Opinion, CNN, November 18, 2020.
[22] "Alison Gopnik on a Revolution to Properly Value Caregivers," *The Economist*, June 18, 2021.

work (see also Ridgeway and Correll 2004, in the context of motherhood) and not viewed as strictly instrumental to society's success. Further development of family allowances, childcare subsidies, parental leave, and even "elder care" leave would help bring the economics of care up to speed with the reality of its necessity.

Gopnik captures how care provides the groundwork for capitalism when she says, "Care expands an individual agent's utilities to include the utilities and goals of another," something Marx's compatriot Engels began discussing 150 years ago. Parents are happier, and disadvantaged children are healthier, in societies with flexible work-family arrangements (Andersson, Garcia, and Glass 2021; Glass, Simon, and Andersson 2016). Among parents, time spent with children is emotionally rewarding (Musick, Meier, and Flood 2016) and avoids the guilt and pangs of time spent *without* children, which is higher in countries with less work flexibility (Berghammer and Milkie 2021). Women's daily hours spent on childcare during the pandemic increased to a level where was close to four times that seen among men.[23] Meanwhile, one in three women globally are victims of intimate partner violence or other sexual violence.[24]

Because parenthood and work both are invested with meaning, they both provide social material for the self. The question as to whether dignity is achieved "despite" opting out really is a question of how individuals relate to and experience major life transitions. A significant sense of loss might set in when one scales back or gets off track relative to one's ambitions (Rao 2021).

Professional mothers in particular face a variety of well-documented backlashes (Ridgeway and Correll 2004). For instance, they can be socially penalized for displays of emotional warmth that normally are invited or even expected among women in general (Cuddy, Fiske, and Glick 2004; Noonan, Lynn, and Walker 2020). In fact, as Noonan and colleagues point out, role expectations associated with being a good or ideal worker directly conflict with those of being a good mother, leading to a "cultural contradiction."

Minority parents are more likely to raise a child alone, compounding the difficulty of being an ideal worker. Also, among two-parent minority households, an accumulation of family and life stressors relative to white

---

[23] "The COVID-19 Pandemic Has Increased the Care Burden, but by How Much?," UN Women Research Highlight: Gender and COVID-19, December 3, 2020. For more on household labor during the initial months of the Covid-19 pandemic, see Carlson, Petts, and Pepin (2021).

[24] "Devastatingly Pervasive: 1 in 3 Women Globally Experience Violence," UN Women, Combating Violence, March 9, 2021.

households intensifies the difficulty of parenting and reinforces racial differences in career success—and in "separate spheres" sexism.

At the same time, of course, the sexism we see in America today is of a different kind and scope than the sexism seen in other nations fighting extremist barriers to human rights. For instance, the Taliban invasion of Afghanistan poses a direct threat not just to life and safety but also to the education and jobs that had served as routes of mobility among Afghan women. Nations with fewer opportunities for women are less economically productive, use more child labor, and have worse public health and lower levels of education.[25] When women rise, societies rise with them, as scores of social demographers, and Melinda Gates (2019), have noted.

Returning to the importance of biological age in American capitalism, its role goes beyond acting as a risk factor for mental or physical disability. Due to the ageism embedded in American worker culture, workers constantly fight the beliefs of others or themselves that they are not what they used to be and that they are "past their prime." Research has shown that negative age stereotypes are applied to the self and in this way can accelerate a loss of cognitive functioning beyond what is observed among individuals who do not apply these stereotypes to themselves (Levy et al. 2009). However, the tricky reality of age stereotyping is that stereotypes are both enacted and internalized, and breaking the cycle depends on a concerted, multifaceted effort among targets and observers alike (Ridgeway 2014, 2019)—brute individual will by itself is unlikely to be enough to keep the stigma completely at bay.

For instance, consider the fact that age stereotyping is for the most part implicit, and many people do not realize that they are negatively evaluating themselves on account of their advanced age. An everyday moment of not remembering a name or fact might be attributed by a young person to lack of sleep or paying attention, whereas older people are more likely to think of their age as an explanation for why they are so forgetful. Other explanations besides age can be far more likely in many situations.

---

[25] "Facts and Figures," Commission on the Status of Women 2012, United Nations Women, https://www.unwomen.org/en/news/in-focus/commission-on-the-status-of-women-2012/facts-and-figures.

## Privatization of Risk: Unequal Chances among America's Children

Privatization of risk is core to defining what American capitalism means and how it is experienced. By this phrase, we do not mean there are no safety nets. Instead, we mean individuals are held responsible for their outcomes in a way that may not be realistic given the economic and social circumstances of American capitalism. Handling life's difficulties is, in the dominant ideology, a matter of self-glory or self-blame. Some individuals face much longer odds when it comes to getting ahead in life, not to mention escaping poverty. One important example is intergenerational social mobility (Chetty et al. 2017). The key trend of declining social mobility within the United States over the past few decades shows that nine of ten children used to outearn their parents; now fewer than one in two achieve this once-expected goal. Meanwhile, about one in twenty can expect to move from poverty to the upper middle class.

Partly as a result of stagnant economic mobility, income inequality within the United States has escalated. The correlated trends of declining mobility and increasing inequality effectively mean that opportunity and wealth are becoming increasingly concentrated in fewer families and fewer communities, reinforced by childhood family structure (Bloome 2017). Meanwhile, communities are becoming increasingly gated by income. All the while, ideologies of self-reliance remain generally strong (Mijs 2018, 2021), as income inequality and individualism go hand in hand. Marx died before capitalism merged with individualistic attributions of success, creating a shiny patina of perceived fairness.

Essentially, meritocracy only leads to social flourishing in the presence of equal and ample opportunity beginning early in life—and in the presence of multiple, diverse criteria of worth (Lamont 2019). Increasingly, as Lamont maintains, America's story is one of unequal opportunity and of fewer criteria of moral worth, adding to a sense of collective unrest. Because academic, social, and emotional skills build rapidly and cumulatively within the first decade of life and are highly shaped by family social class—and by the schools, neighborhoods, and communities that transmit these class effects—the notion of meritocracy becomes veiled classism, and a neoliberal tendency to hold individuals responsible for their efforts begins to look like holding them responsible for birth lots (Hall and Lamont 2013; Markovits

2019). Meanwhile, living within this system worsens our ability to see its true workings, limiting our sociological imagination.

Early divergences in cognitive, emotional, and social development by family social class widen from infancy to childhood (Heckman 2006; Jackson 2015; Kuh and Shlomo 2004; Masten and Cicchetti 2010; Mayer 2009). Of course, families can move school districts or can improve their economic situations, but these turn out to be relatively uncommon deviations at the population level. Whether a child attends college—and, just as important, where they attend—serves as a vital link in preventing downward economic mobility and increasing odds of upward mobility. Career funneling into high-paying fields such as finance, business, science, and engineering occurs disproportionately from selective or elite colleges (Binder, Davis, and Bloom 2016). As ethnographic research by the sociologist Amy Binder has shown, the career interests that students declare on their personal statements are refashioned into the careers that students "should" desire—while working for a nongovernmental organization (NGO) perhaps sounds appealing when entering an elite school, working in consulting becomes deemed more practical, realistic, or lucrative. For many years, Ivy League graduates have commonly placed into finance or consulting positions at Goldman Sachs or McKinsey, for instance, and these kinds of placements become more common as a university becomes more elite.[26]

Beyond the brute facts about declining mobility and increasing in-equality, the United States has staggering rates of poverty compared to its peers. Not treating housing as a right or treating housing as a set of precarious entitlements that do not rule out eviction or dislocation (Desmond 2012) creates a situation where having a home cannot be taken for granted, especially among the poor. Health care, while subsidized through programs such as Medicaid, is a complex patchwork that takes tremendous time, energy, and discretionary income to successfully navigate, especially for treatments of major or life-threatening diseases. As a result, whether Medicaid reduces poverty turns out to be contingent on the particulars of one's health situation and on state-level expansions (Zewde and Wimer 2019). Food insecurity, economic strain, and unsafe living conditions disproportionately associated with poverty are added, separate sources of stress (e.g., Mirowsky and Ross 1999; Seligman and Berkowitz 2019).

---

[26] Jonathan Zimmerman, "Our Best and Brightest Bankers," *Chronicle of Higher Education*, July 9, 2018.

Once housing, food, transportation, childcare, utilities, and other routine expenses are considered, many Americans' economic margins are razor thin or negative, leading to chronic economic stress. Autonomy, poise, self-sufficiency, freedom from stigma, safety, nutrition, education, and planning for a future for oneself and one's family all have been proposed ingredients in the achievement of dignity in America, and all are made more difficult by poverty, making poverty itself arguably a structural measure of chronic indignity as individuals live on the margins.

In studying unhoused individuals, Snow and Anderson (1987) made the symbolic interactionist argument, later to be extended, that one can draw moral distinctions between oneself and the society and people who are resourced and, in this way, preserve a sense of personal dignity. But this sort of dignity is likely to be far less sustaining than that afforded by an absence of social and economic marginalization in the first place. The poor are disproportionately people of color. As the sociologist Elijah Anderson (2022) documents in *Black in White Space: The Enduring Impact of Color in Everyday Life*, society is composed predominantly of white-owned and white-occupied spaces: to work and to live, Black people enter these white spaces. Due to discrimination or a sense of exclusion, Blacks suffer an enduring sense of not being at home in society.

## College Attendance and Graduation: Implications of Racism and Racial Inequality

Given these stark differences in outcomes and living conditions, many of which are linked with some significance to obtaining a college degree, who actually goes to college, where do they matriculate, and who graduates? Family socioeconomic status matters significantly to admission, and to the supposedly neutral standardized test scores shaping it (Alon and Tienda 2007; Hearn 1991). While personal statements on college applications prize student resilience, actual admissions rates usually do not reflect the degree of difficulty people had on their paths toward college. Selective and elite schools continue to screen on other, class-related characteristics such as academic interests, student grade point average or achievement, or extracurricular accomplishments (Farkas 2018; Lucas 2001, 2009).

This is hardly to say that colleges should ignore all this information, but rather that it highlights what sociologists and economists of education have known for a long time. Namely, the association between family social class and attendance at a selective school—or any four-year college—is multifaceted and begins even before birth, with maternal health and family stress, and continues after birth through toddler word gaps, early reading and math achievement, preschool enrollment, and other early steps, all eventually translating into primary and secondary school achievement (Ansari and Pianta 2018; Hanushek 2009; Heckman and Krueger 2003; Jackson 2015). Attendance at a two-year college, graduation from a two-year college, and transfer to a four-year college all are patterned by family social class (Schudde and Brown 2019).

Meanwhile, the divide in who attends and graduates from college reinforces a variety of inequalities in society, in particular racial inequality because of how race and class are profoundly correlated: segregation, wealth gaps, and primary and second school resources, among other processes, induce this correlation. Even more, class hardly stands in for race, as minority children sustain lower-quality schools, less safe neighborhoods, and greater stress even when their levels of income or education are the same as their white counterparts (Williams 2018; Williams and Mohammed 2013).

American primary and secondary schools operate at the nexus of class and race (Reardon, Kalogrides, and Shores 2019) by enrolling students in ways delineated by residential situation. As is well documented by urban sociologists, residential segregation by race is modestly—not greatly—lower than it was decades ago and is virtually unchanged for many metropolitan statistical areas (MSAs) across the United States. School quality—in terms of per-student funding, student performance, teacher-to-student ratios, or teacher ability and pay, for instance—is much greater for predominantly white school districts compared to majority-minority districts. In fact, during the Covid-19 pandemic, the U.S. Department of Education reinitiated collection of school civil rights data to document how schooling inequalities worsened by the pandemic might also lead to widening racial and ethnic educational achievement gaps they feared would grow and persist long after the pandemic begins to abate.

Racial inequalities in the educational process stem not just from public schools of widely varying college-preparatory quality, but also from other pernicious links, such as the "school-to-prison pipeline," capturing how lower-quality schools set up minority students to fail out and become much more likely to be incarcerated.[27] In a recent feature for *The Atlantic,* Harvard

---

[27] "The School-to-Prison Pipeline, Explained," Vox.com, October 27, 2015.

sociologist Bruce Western drew on decades of incarceration data and the sociologist Devah Pager's well-known research into incarceration and labor market outcomes (e.g., Pager and Shepherd 2008; Quillian et al. 2017) to reveal interconnections among parental incarceration, parental hardship, children's education, and racial inequalities in incarceration.[28] What we learn from this research is that American school systems create great opportunity while also creating limited opportunities for those who do not attend higher-quality schools and who do not finish high school or attend college, and that completing high school is linked to parental and family resources. Our legal system as it operates has produced more and longer sentences for minoritized groups including Blacks and Latinos, even when presumptive sentences, criminal history, and other background characteristics are controlled (Alexander 2011; King and Johnson 2016).[29]

## Sexism and Educational and Occupational Achievement

While women have outpaced men since the 1980s in earning bachelor's degrees (DiPrete and Buchmann 2013), the fields of these degrees segregated by gender, as does the receipt of master's and doctoral degrees in many lucrative fields (DiPrete and Buchmann 2013; Legewie and DiPrete 2014; Montez et al. 2018). Another core result of education is an improved sense of control. Although education enhances the sense of control similarly by gender, women's mental health may benefit more from a sense of control than men's (Ross, Masters, and Hummer 2012). However, economic and occupational educational returns such as labor force participation, earnings, authority, job satisfaction, and occupational prestige—and avoidance of gender discrimination more generally—are overall more favorable for men (Andersson and Harnois 2020; Pudrovska 2013; Pudrovska and Karraker 2014; Roscigno, Yavorsky, and Quadlin 2021). Moreover, the authority associated with higher-status jobs is disproportionately burdensome on women's health, in part due to the greater amount of emotional and logistical labor involved compared to men holding authority positions (Pudrovska and Karraker

[28] "The Racism of Mass Incarceration, Visualized," *The Atlantic*, September 11, 2015.
[29] See also Michelle Alexander's (2011) *The New Jim Crow: Mass Incarceration in the Age of Colorblindness*.

2014) and likely also due to the greater structural incompatibility between work and family among women (Montez et al. 2014; Rao 2021).

For instance, science, technology, engineering, and math disciplines systemically attenuate women more than men at most stages of educational and career pipelines associated with these disciplines (Cech and Blair-Loy 2010; Correll 2004; Sassler et al. 2017); the related discipline of medicine remains predominantly male, as do most pockets of law, business, management, and finance (Tomaskovic-Devey and Skaggs 2002).

Going to college often means taking on considerable debt, though less debt for students from more advantaged families (Houle 2014). The effects of this debt burden are unequal by race, in part due to differences in types of schools attended and lines of credit extended (Seamster and Charron-Chénier 2017) and gender, because economic and social returns to college are lower among racial and ethnic minorities (Williams and Mohammed 2013) and among women (England 2010). Even with a recent U.S. Department of Education decision to cancel some forms of student debt, and even with Target, Starbucks, and other employers offering to foot the bill for some university educations, the larger, looming question as to who should pay for college persists. From 2010 to 2019, public sentiment has shifted toward a much-increased preference for government funding (Quadlin and Powell 2022).

## Conclusion: Meritocracy as Structural Indignity

A perceived meritocracy rewarding hard work and talent invigorates and empowers. The version we live with in America, however, calcifies inequality by inciting apathy to social structure, through this same fixation on individual uniqueness. Classism, ableism, sexism, racism, and ageism written into capitalism's interlinked, massive structures all become harder to see and harder to change. Rigid visions of merit presume resourced situations while appearing to do exactly the opposite. We say "valuing hard work" when what we really mean is the opportunity and ability to work exceptionally, both of which stem from abundant capital and positional advantages. Dignity's basis in social appreciation and meaningful work is at stake in American capitalism.

# 5

# Measuring Dignity Subjectively

## Methodology for 2017 and 2021 Gallup Data

In the coming chapters, we measure dignity subjectively, in terms of whether people perceive or experience "dignity" within their own lives. By measuring these individual dignity perceptions, we can examine patterns of experienced dignity across different groups, social classes, and other forms of categorization in America. To paraphrase Sir Michael Marmot (2004), this could lend new insight into whether we are achieving dignity, and for whom.

While numerical measurement of dignity might be dismissed as a reduction of personhood to statistics, we make an overarching case here and in the coming chapters as well that the benefits of measuring dignity probably outweigh any costs or shortcomings. Andrew Sayer (2011, 191) similarly alludes to the promise of a science of dignity: "If we examine it, and what secures or threatens it, it reveals much about our relation to the world of concern." In the coming chapters, we want to demonstrate how dignity can be an efficient indicator for wider social processes and explore what it tells us about American society both before and during the 2019 pandemic, and how dignity can inform health research for decades to come.

Class, gender, and racial inequalities all bear relevance to dignity, for example, at least theoretically (Hodson 1996; Lamont 2000; Oeur 2016; Sayer 2011; Silva 2013). How, exactly, are perceptions of dignity patterned by these axes of social inequality, as outlined in Chapter 4? That is, rather than simply examining structural conditions surrounding dignity, how can we link those same structures to experiences of and perspectives on dignity per se (Hitlin and Andersson 2013), and what can that tell us about how modern society both reflects and reproduces social inequalities? We cannot put a price on dignity, but we can quantify how much dignity people believe they have, and thereby provide a new way of bringing social personhood—and the moral

*The Science of Dignity.* Steven Hitlin and Matthew A. Andersson, Oxford University Press.
© Oxford University Press 2023. DOI: 10.1093/oso/9780197743867.003.0006

and complexity it entails—into conversations about population health (Hitlin and Andersson 2015).

Following many scholars, if we were to assume that dignity equates to autonomy or a sense of control over one's life, or to recognition and respect within one's community, we might then go about measuring dignity using these established indicators that presumably capture its key aspects. Similarly, if we were taking a human rights approach to dignity, it would make good sense to think of—and measure—dignity in terms of violence, humiliation, abuse, exploitation, or other commonly recognized violations of humanity. Enslavement and human trafficking also figure prominently in human rights discussions. For instance, "human trafficking is an unconscionable attack on the dignity of the most vulnerable among us," as President Biden noted. As other examples, a Patient Dignity Inventory draws on autonomy and quality-of-life-related concepts among cancer patients (Xiao et al. 2019), and qualitative research shows "the significance of small things for dignity" in psychiatric care (Skorpen, Rehnsfeldt, and Thorsen 2015).

Building on this clinical scholarship, as well as a sociological tradition of dignity research, we show in the coming chapters how dignity might mean even more to America, in ways that both reflect and extend these applied applications in the hospital or in the workplace, for example. *Dignity within a life both incorporates and supersedes social particularities.* It encapsulates a presence of resources for identity as well as an absence of overt or systemic threats to life. As we analyze it here, "dignity" could serve as a subjective measurement strategy that usefully adds to existing research on particular social problems such as structural injustice, job precarity, poverty, stigma, health care quality, and abuse or neglect.

## Looking for a Gold Standard: Positing Criteria for Efficient Indication of Complex Social Processes

What kind of stock should we place in a measure of subjective dignity? What does variation in individual dignity perceptions mean, and how should we interpret it? In the coming chapters, we will be building a case for dignity as an encompassing yet parsimonious measure of social and moral integration in America. In building our case, it might help to provide an overview of other comprehensive, subjective measures used by social scientists and epidemiologists. We do so by briefly discussing their properties, and whether those same properties might be expected to hold for the measurement of subjective dignity that we will utilize.

First, we consider a gold standard measure that has been used in public health, epidemiology, and clinical medicine for decades. Referred to as self-rated health (e.g., Idler and Benyamini 1997; Jylhä 2009), the measure asks the reader to rate their health, from poor to excellent (Figure 5.1).

Self-rated health is, of course, subjective: people are reporting on their own perceived, overall health, and they might have differing thresholds for thinking about what "excellent" or "poor" health looks or feels like. Also, the measure does not refer to objective diseases or specific health problems, aiming instead for a general, personal assessment of health. Respondents understand it in numerous ways correlated with actual health outcomes, even if they would be unable to explain precisely how or why.

In view of—and perhaps "despite"—these properties, self-rated health has been shown to predict longevity and quality of life, while also significantly associating with myriad objective health problems or their severity (Idler and Cartwright 2018). In fact, self-rated health predicts future well-being *net* of an extensive checklist of medical information.

Why is self-rated health a gold standard among epidemiologists and physicians alike? Perhaps because it captures so much so efficiently: it takes the massive complexity of a health interview and winnows it down to a single, straightforward question that can be used for effective triaging or outcome prediction.

As it turns out, where one places oneself from "excellent" to "poor" on self-rated health reflects a social understanding of a variety of diagnosed and undiagnosed diseases as well as present and past experiences of illness and symptoms. It also captures the intersection of cultural beliefs about illness and local health comparisons with others that could matter for feelings of self-worth. If individuals are currently experiencing any overwhelming health difficulties, this question would capture that as well. *The aim is not perfection of measurement, but rather meaningfulness and capacity of measurement.* Self-rated health *adds* useful information to the summarization of

> "In general, would you say your health is:
> □ Excellent □ Very Good □ Good □ Fair □ Poor"

**Figure 5.1**  A Typical Survey Question for Self-Rated Health

health, but it does not *replace* objective, clinical information that would be useful to follow up on and figure out what to do next.

Similarly, with the measurement of subjective dignity, we might hope to glean an overall sense of dignity before zooming in on the particulars of what might be shaping or influencing that dignity. As we have shown, dignity generally has a "good news" distribution in America: most people believe they have a good deal of it. Similarly, self-rated health distributions tend to be favorably skewed, with most people reporting "good," "very good," or "excellent" health. Still, epidemiologists often focus on "fair" or "poor" responses to the self-rated health item, as these lower categories can be especially potent when it comes to isolating those with major or life-threatening health concerns. Similarly, we have already highlighted how health and well-being are especially lower for those experiencing dignity threat.

To be sure, just because most people report good or excellent self-rated health does not mean that health problems are not a societal concern. In the United States, we have higher rates of cancer, heart disease, and obesity and lower life expectancy than we should have based on our national level of economic development. Similarly, the fact that most people report a generally positive sense of dignity does not represent an absence of indignity in society. We are additionally troubled by the finding that from 2017 to 2021, the number of individuals placing themselves in the lowermost categories of dignity essentially doubled.

Decades ago, how did leading scholars working in public health, epidemiology, and medicine go about convincing their colleagues that a self-rated health measure could be worthwhile and useful? Researchers advocating the measure needed criteria to make their case. By gathering extensive indices of symptoms, disease, and general sickness, they were able to show two key things: (1) the self-rated health measure powerfully predicted differences in objective health criteria, and (2) self-rated health could predict future health above and beyond the information provided by objective health checklists or laboratory tests, suggesting that self-rated health taps into bodily, vitality, or somatic information that might fall through the cracks of clinical checklists—or even evade blood test results. This subjective indicator efficiently captures important information useful to population health research in America; perhaps dignity can serve a similar diagnostic role.

## Another Gold Standard: Subjective Social Status

About two decades ago, a new, streamlined measure of socioeconomic status began gaining traction among health psychologists and then diffused with great success to other disciplines including public health and sociology (Adler et al. 2000). This measure, termed "subjective social status," involves having individuals rank themselves based on where they think they stand within society's socioeconomic hierarchy. Decades of research had found that educational level, income, and occupational resources predict depression, illness, and death with surprising power, but plenty of error still was present in these predictions, and researchers were looking for ways to gain more insight into how it is that social class influences health (Adler and Tan 2017; Andersson 2018a; Cundiff and Matthews 2017).

Consider the example of a subjective social status measure, taken from our 2017 Gallup survey, shown in Figure 5.2. Here, people are asked whether they consider themselves "worst off," "about average," "best off," or something else in between relative to the reference groups of "other Americans," neighbors, or friends. The subjective social status question mentions "money, education, and a good job" as the general bases of comparison. As it turns out, much of how social class operates in society is *relative* and *subjective* (Andersson 2022; Schnittker and McLeod 2005): that is, how individuals understand and live their social position stems from how they are situated in their communities, where they think they stand within hierarchies, and how they think about the larger society they live in. The perceptions are experienced as practical facts that are as important as the actual facts, many of which people are unaware of or do not interpret in the same way.

---

"In terms of having money, education, and a good job,

how do you compare to other Americans?"

0 (worst off) ..1..2..3..4..5 (about average) ..6..7..8..9..10 (best off)

---

**Figure 5.2**  A Typical Survey Question for Subjective Social Status

## Subjective Measurement: Limitations Pale in Comparison to Gained Information

Just like any measure, subjective measures are imperfect and incomplete: people's perceptions may or may not reflect their actual situations. However, people generally do not exhibit denialism: for instance, poverty and financial strain usually are jointly subjective and objective realities (e.g., Shuey and Willson 2014). Given this fact, we can benefit from the massive amount of information that subjective assessments can tap without us needing to ask an exhaustive—and limited or predefined—set of questions. Indeed, subjective understandings are socially constructed based on individual socialization, reference groups, motivations, and communities, and to neglect this fact would be to deny individuals the possibility of social intelligence. To paraphrase W. I. and Dorothy Thomas (1928), if a person believes something to be real, it is real in its consequences.

## Revisiting the Quantification Critique: Do Dignity Numbers Numb Us to Dignity Itself?

One might object to subjective dignity by saying that dignity is desecrated or destroyed through measurement of "superficial" dignity perceptions. That is, by creating a dignity scale, we ironically transform unique lives into one-dimensional numbers, in dignity's name. For example, two survey respondents each scoring 75% on a dignity scale are, effectively speaking, equalized with regard to dignity, at least in terms of statistical analysis. To return to Kant's foundational insight, lives—by definition—cannot be measured against each other.

Following Kant: If dignity is "without price," does that mean it is without quantification? We think not. Because of the sacralization of individuality that modern dignity implies, individuals themselves become theory-generating entities for dignity. As long as we remember that identical dignity scores do not mean identical life circumstances, the pursuit is quite fruitful. Similarly, two people who both have "good" self-rated health likely have quite different experiences and biographies of their bodies and minds. This measurement property is omnipresent within social science and is referred to as *equifinality*: that is, multiple or numerous paths to the same numeric outcome level (see also Ragin 1999).

The sociologist John Levi Martin (2011, ix) proposes that "because we have not trusted the social world to have its own principles of regularity, we have forced our theories to have this regularity 'prefabricated.'" Perhaps in the case of dignity, we might need to pull back on the prefabrication, instead favoring a more localized approach to individual meaning making.

Certainly, the preceding chapters might be used to argue that dignity has objective roots in material and economic conditions, and therefore necessitates an objective measurement strategy. However, as we also took care to develop, the objective conditions set a stage for, but do not determine, particularized, subjective realizations and understandings of dignity at the lived intersection of multiple networks, commitments, hierarchies, beliefs, and identities. Dignity thus may represent an instance where social theory and individuality dissolve each other (Giddens 1991). Dignity incorporates—in a literal, corporeal sense—social structures, while also rejecting them through lived particularities.

Quantification collapses and, on some level, destroys much experiential information about being in the world. Embodiment and situation, as two crowning conceits of sociological science, elude a strict logic of numbers so familiar to quantitative social scientists (e.g., Wacquant 2014). A notion of dignity suggests a possibility to quantify humanity but not necessarily what specifically matters within individual lives.

Beginning at least with William James, social psychologists confronted a similar conceptual issue when converting "the self" into an empirical research program. Since then, prized concepts such as self-esteem and identity have become a basis not only of understanding well-being but also of the public's imagination of itself: people have literally come to perform and enact the science of self-esteem through the controversial, profitable advent of the self-help genre, not to mention mental health TikToks.

Even if dignity is experienced differently across individuals, this does not mean it cannot or should not be studied scientifically. Distinct social patterns exist, even in our most personal, authentic selves (e.g., Turner 1976; Turner and Schutte 1981). Personality is an example of a scientific area of inquiry that is furthered by the development of traits, taxonomies, and other ways of understanding *between*-individual consistencies that shed some light on *within*-individual situational experiences, even while no two personalities are precisely the same. Indeed, the study of personality is subject to nomothetic approaches, which emphasize the derivation of principles, and idiographic approaches, which emphasize the particularized manifestations of personalities in individual lives (Mischel and Shoda 1995).

In the same way, dignity might be approached from both sides: in terms of its cross-individual patterns and within-individual, subjective construction of situations. How we might talk about dignity draws on a moral repertoire or set of relevant vocabularies that changes over time (Lamont and Thévenot 2000; Lakoff and Johnson 1999). By querying "dignity" directly, we instantiate value neutrality about what dignity might mean either within or across specific situations, allowing subjects to read in their own, variable definitions of the concept.

Dignity, like morality itself, has a plurality of definitions or conceptions that are considerably situation dependent. Maintaining one's dignity in the face of an oppressive society, as members of many minority racial and sexual orientation groups do, is not quite the same as maintaining dignity while being fired, or in a military occupation, or in spilling one's food at dinner. However—and crucially, for the approach to dignity we take here—this situationism would not preclude the value of subjective assessments cutting across situations, as these assessments also allow for the subjective possibility of a plurality of definitions, and how individuals imbue import to these dynamic definitions and their interrelationships. Put simply, individuals differently give weight to their experiences and their various interpretations.

Mastery or a sense of control is one of the most measured psychological resources (Mirowsky and Ross 2007; Pearlin and Bierman 2013): what makes one feel empowered in one situation is not the same as in another, and yet individuals are asked, usefully, by surveys to rate their overall sense of control across the various problems they are confronting in their lives. People feel differently about themselves in different roles—you might feel positive about your dancing ability but negative about your ability to make friends. Both get grouped under a general measure of "self-esteem," although domain-specific self-esteem or self-efficacy can be measured when useful (e.g., Bandura 1977; Rosenberg et al. 1995; Shelton 1990). Dignity measurement, we believe, could operate on a similar basic premise, in which individuals appraise their own lived lives from a bird's-eye view, seeing or perceiving dignity patterns from on high, across all situations big and small shaping their own dignity.

As we discuss in the next chapter, measures of perceived discrimination also have usefully focused on the actor's view instead of the observer's (Major, Dovidio, and Link 2018; Monk 2021; Pascoe and Richman 2009), from the standpoint of understanding patterns of subjective and physiological distress and thereby understanding long-term physical health outcomes such as hypertension, disease, and death.

*Our analysis of Gallup data focuses on cross-individual patterns of dignity and what they might teach us about how societies and individuals relate.* Is dignity something that you know about yourself, or is it something others rate about you? In focusing on subjective appraisals of *one's own* dignity, we elide examination of how we view *each other's* dignity or lack thereof. We might hold that autonomy is the core of dignity, while a different set of scholars or a different culture might focus on self-worth or freedom from discrimination, while a third culture might prize masculinity or grit. By steering clear of preidentified conceptions of dignity, we acknowledge the dynamism and plurality of dignity across individual lives.

While we will be tracking trends and associations related to dignity to glean insights *across* people, less clear is whether people *think* about dignity in similar ways. However, even without this evidence, we still find that dignity associates with respect, perceived discrimination, resources, stress, and socioeconomic status, to name a few examples, leading us to conclude that how people think about dignity does in fact demonstrate some noticeable patterns, even without knowing which particular conceptions of dignity particular individuals might mobilize and for which particular social situations (e.g., Goffman 1963; Lamont et al. 2016; Lizardo 2017; Swidler 2001).

At least three empirically relevant questions arise once one thinks seriously about dignity's existence in the social world (following Brennan and Lo 2007): (1) Does dignity vary between people? (2) If dignity does vary across individuals, then how should we treat or think about people who possess differing degrees of dignity? and (3) What merits or qualities are dignity relevant?

The first question might be called the variational question. We engage this beginning in Chapter 6. From the perspective of intrinsic dignity, dignity is a brute fact of being human, and no real variation should exist, at least at the level of political rhetoric and legal theory. However, from the perspective of recognized or attributed dignity, it could make sense to see individuals as thinking of themselves as possessing varying degrees of dignity based on the differing degrees of adversity or stress they confront, or their differing networks, beliefs, or coping resources, for example. Insofar as we think of dignity as something that can change over time, or be wounded by social circumstance, it could vary.

The second question is morally prescriptive in nature. From the standpoint of population health science, we can designate health or well-being as a *criterion* against which to ascertain whether declines in a subjective sense of dignity "matter": whether they are linked to differences in physical or mental flourishing, or in depression, illness, or bodily inflammation or stress, and if so, use these health inequalities as a moral warrant for redressing these perceived dignity differences.[1]

The third question gets to the crux of many of our analyses. In the ensuing chapters, people will report how much dignity they feel, and as we will demonstrate, its associations with respect, perceived discrimination, health, resources, inequality, and stress show important patterns.[2]

Ultimately, across these analytic questions, we find that dignity is correlated with a variety of important social and health-related phenomena without being interchangeable with any of them. This is what we might hope for when building an initial case for an efficient, encompassing indicator of social and moral personhood, which we might find in dignity.

Our business for the remaining chapters follows the philosopher of science Michael Streven's "iron rule of explanation":[3] if scientists "are to participate in the scientific enterprise, they must uncover or generate new evidence to argue with." In other words, our goal is to offer new data that sheds additional light on how dignity works, who thinks they have it, and dignity's social consequences. As our reader is generously aware, a main purpose of this book is to offer preliminary, criterion-based evidence for subjective dignity's importance, by comparing across known social groups and hierarchies and their structural adversities, and by bringing in conventional measures of health and well-being.

We cannot offer a conclusive case that dignity makes an optimal or seamless transition from the conceptual realm to the empirical realm, a standard

[1] Perhaps pure neutrality about studying human beings would not judge being healthier as "better," given the inherent value judgment. This can (and has) led to a rabbit hole of debate over the rights of researchers to impose their own values or priorities onto the people they are studying; perhaps some groups do not want democracy, or technology, or other "advances" that can be studied. We are dodging this issue, suggesting that better health is an a priori good, and thus examining what health is related to as a worthwhile empirical exercise.

[2] Elsewhere we have speculative quantitative measures of dignity's properties; in later chapters, we will show how dignity measures get us something beyond the other putative aspects, like self-esteem or mastery.

[3] From Joshua Rathman, "How Does Science Really Work?," *New Yorker*, September 28, 2020. Thank you to Lynn Smith-Lovin for referencing this piece during her remarks to the social psychology section at the 2021 American Sociological Association annual meeting.

that, in our opinion, only can be met through cumulative scientific efforts across scholars. Documenting correlations between "dignity" as measured and health does not mean that we have taken a true road to measuring dignity itself. This point cannot be overemphasized. As a statistician might say, a true model of social processes cannot be determined given observed data, only whether a model is not rejected given observed data. Importantly, this implies that other approaches to dignity measurement or to testing statistical associations taken by authors in future research could also be shown to be not-false and, like ours, never definitively true.[4] As social pragmatists, the question we might ask is, "are these strategies useful, and how?"

Working through a subjectivist lens, we believe that dignity perceptions contribute significantly to the study of social order: dignity provides a long-awaited measure of perceptions of living up to moral standards that, for the most part, avoids the conceptual morass of *which* moral standards across a polarized American society and even across situations and times within individual lives (Hitlin and Vaisey 2013; Luft 2020). Because dignity embraces—and indeed incorporates—the complex idiosyncrasies of how individuality interfaces with society, it might help circumvent some longstanding debates in the study of morality and the social. Dignity gives a rare opportunity to study morality holistically and individualistically—and, of course, in a socially meaningful way.

## Our Subjective Dignity Measure: Subjectively Defining the Objectively Undefinable

For the remaining chapters, we draw on repeated cross-sectional, national survey data collected by Gallup in 2017 and again in 2021, as part of the Values and Beliefs of the American Public Survey. In the 2017 and 2021 surveys, subjective dignity is measured by self-reported perceptions of dignity in one's own life. This survey offers a random sample of adults aged eighteen and older, living in all fifth U.S. states and the District of Columbia. In February 2017, Gallup randomly selected individuals to participate using an address-based sample (ABS) frame, mailing eleven thousand surveys with

---

[4] We are simply pointing this out for accuracy's sake. Many philosophical tracts get into the nature of knowledge in science; we leave those to the enterprising reader.

Gallup 2017 Values and Beliefs of the American Public Survey

*Subjective Dignity Survey Items*

"I feel that my life lacks dignity."*
"I have dignity as a person."
"People generally treat me with dignity."*
"People generally are not respectful toward me."
"My dignity is not up to me."
"I determine my own dignity."*

*Asked in 2017 and 2021 Surveys

For each question above, the response options were:

□ Strongly Disagree    □ Disagree    □ Agree    □ Strongly Agree    □ Undecided

**Figure 5.3**  Survey Questions for Subjective Dignity (from 2017 and 2021 Gallup Surveys)

a one-dollar cash incentive, with reminder postcards following about two weeks later. The collection of completed interviews ended on March 21, with $n = 1,501$. In 2021, surveys were sent to a separate, random ABS frame sample of eleven thousand households. Respondents were allowed to respond to the survey on paper or via the web. The survey was conducted from January 27 to March 21, in English and Spanish ($n = 1,248$).

Across the six related items, "dignity" is mentioned in all but one, which instead mentions "respect" (Figure 5.3).

We do not include "respect" in our measure of subjective dignity for five main reasons: (1) a subjective dignity measure is easier to understand as such when it focuses on "dignity" as a term; (2) a five-item dignity measure, excluding "respect," shows adequate fit in indicating an overall dignity factor; (3) the general conclusions we present in the coming chapters regarding morality, health, resources, and stress are unchanged regardless of this decision; (4) excluding the "respect" item allows us to validate our measure in the next chapter of the book, since "respect" is an often-mentioned synonym of dignity; and (5) in comparing dignity levels from 2017 to 2021, we are restricted to the three items used across both years.

For all analyses in the remaining chapters, we form a scale across these three items, which involves taking the average response across all three items. "I feel that my life lacks dignity," "People generally treat me with dignity," and "I determine my own dignity" were used in both years (denoted in Figure 5.3

by an asterisk), allowing for the construction of a three-item scale that we can use to compare dignity levels from 2017 to 2021.[5]

Our choice to use a subjective dignity *scale* rather than individual dignity items for most of the analyses we present reflects four main considerations: (1) exploratory and confirmatory factor models generally support the use of a scale; (2) using a scale keeps our presentation far more streamlined and manageable; (3) the scale, as a holistic tool, comes closer to achieving our theoretical objective of flexible dignity definitions, because dignity is used in multiple senses across these items; and (4) explicating dignity in terms of different dignity items is more suited to formal scale development, which would likely involve starting with a much larger pool of potential items.[6]

## What Does Subjective Dignity Measure?

In social science, it is typical to assess whether something—a concept of some kind—matters by showing what it predicts. That is the general approach we take across the remaining chapters. We begin in Chapter 6 with a set of concepts theoretically related to dignity that, according to many scholars, could be part of how dignity arises. While we unfortunately cannot offer an exhaustive treatment, the closely related concepts we are able to examine using the Gallup data include morality, respect, perceived discrimination, lack of severe economic disadvantage, autonomy, mastery, mattering to others, and having some sense of meaning in life. While few scholars would

---

[5] To offer slightly more detail regarding scale construction in 2017, we used all five items in 2017 to assess the proposed subjective dignity construct, because using only three items does not allow any degrees of freedom for global fit testing of a confirmatory factor model. These items vary in the degree to which they characterize dignity as coming from within rather than without (i.e., "dignity-of-self" and "dignity-in-relation"; Jacobson 2007), so we began with an exploratory factor analysis. In 2017, principal components exploratory factor analysis identified one factor with eigenvalue = 1.688 (factor 2 eigenvalue = 0.144). All factor loadings ranged from 0.42 to 0.71. Confirmatory factor analysis with asymptotically distribution free (ADF) estimation to address response non-normality and free covariances among conceptually similar items retained a one-factor solution against the observed covariance-variance matrix, $\chi^2(2) = 1.663$, $p = .44$, RMSEA = 0.000, CFI = 1.000, TLI = 1.008, SRMR = 0.011. Having established that a one-factor model was consistent with the observed data in 2017, we proceeded to treat all items as belonging to the same subjective dignity scale across both survey years. Specifically, we used the three items available across both survey years for all analyses in this book. Latent factor scores were generated and normalized across both years using Stata 17.0. In 2017, the three-item latent score correlates highly with the five-item latent score ($r = .900$). A polychoric correlation matrix for the five items in 2017 shows a mean intercorrelation of .478.

[6] While our survey contract with Gallup did not allow us to field a larger number of prospective dignity items useful for scale development, future research building on the initial findings here should aim to parse out any effects of distinct types of subjective dignity.

contend that these concepts are interchangeable with dignity, these concepts nonetheless offer concrete guideposts against which to measure whether subjective dignity is measuring what we might think it should measure.

Or, to state the case negatively, a subjective dignity measure might not be viewed as tapping a useful conception of dignity if it did not correlate somewhat strongly with these conceptually related guideposts. The broad argument of Chapter 6, therefore, will be empirical: that dignity carries promise as an efficient indicator of moral and social integration because it correlates strongly and as expected with these related but ultimately different concepts. Meanwhile—and equally crucially—it is not too strongly correlated with any one of them, building a case that dignity is *not* effectively synonymous with what many critics of the concept have contended might be substitutable or "equally good" synonyms. That is, our subjective dignity measure behaves as a distinct indicator.

Like self-rated health and subjective social status, two "gold standard measures" in the epidemiology literature for tapping overall health and overall social status, respectively, subjective dignity has many, varied predictors, and it correlates more strongly with the predictors that come closer to the core of more popular conceptions of dignity. Likewise, self-rated health correlates quite significantly with objective indices of symptoms, disease, and death (e.g., Idler and Benyamini 1997; Jylhä 2009), while subjective social status correlates at considerable magnitudes with objective socioeconomic indicators like education, income, and occupation (Andersson 2018a; Cundiff and Matthews 2017).

So, if subjective dignity correlates with related moral or social concepts but is not interchangeable with these concepts, then what does a measured level of subjective dignity represent? Similarly, researchers of self-rated health offer a detailed list of the various subjective, evaluative, perceptive, bodily, and health processes that self-rated health might be capturing, on some level, in specific social, historical, or cultural situations (Jylhä 2009). In this same vein, our organizing or interpretational framework for these numerous subjective dignity findings specifies that subjective dignity must (1) remain flexible to group-specific or pluralistic senses of the term and (2) remain flexible to the possibility that observed, group-specific levels of dignity reflect (a) objective social conditions, (b) subjective interpretations of these same conditions, and/or (c) socially constructed, possibly dynamic understandings of what dignity means, in ways that are individually or collectively affirming or strategic.

In the ensuing chapters, therefore, we try to be careful about any over-reach in reading too specifically into the quantification of dignity we observe. All claims about group-specific determinants or logics of dignity should be substantiated either by referring to qualitative research on the topic or by future research that charts out these mechanisms more clearly, much of which we have discussed previously.

Beyond the conceptual fact that groups differ in norms, resources, and cultural strategies, we mobilize capitalism as an organizing framework for appreciating group positionality across material hierarchies. Group-based distinctions and legal rights are deeply, historically entwined with capitalism and its differential prioritization of individual lives. Thus, by singling out structural and interpersonal biases attached to sex, race, age, class, and worker status, we provide a richer motivation for how each of these subgroups is situated differently in society and thereby might approach the concept of dignity differently and experience differing levels, following Michèle Lamont's extensive work on this topic.

## Our Descriptive, Cross-Sectional Approach to Dignity and Some of Its Limitations

Our analytic approach here is descriptive. We are asking the straightforward question of what levels of dignity look like across different segments of society, in ways that might spur future research focused on careful statistical or causal inference.[7]

Our analyses are somewhat limited by their cross-sectional nature. Namely, while we track differences in dignity across 2017 and 2021, we surveyed different people in each of these two years, so we cannot make any claims about how dignity changes within individual lives or about individual development across the pandemic. Instead, we rely on broad trends that we track across groups of people to begin to understand what changing dignity might look like and the effects it might have in society. Taken at the population level, we

---

[7] A multivariate approach, which involves adjusting for a variety of demographic factors all at once, ultimately would mask what we want to show, because it is structured around principles of average or net effects across an entire population, which do not interest us here. These population-wide estimates are driven disproportionately by groups with larger sample representation, so we decided against it. Elsewhere, we present these adjusted estimates and tests of statistical significance, and we find strong associations between subjective dignity and self-reported mental and physical health across a variety of demographic groups (Andersson and Hitlin 2022).

suggest it is an efficient indicator of several social trends and pressures. At the individual level, dignity is subject to these broader pressures as well as individual experiences and interpretations.

Overall, we emphasize the predictive value of dignity for health, by showing how incremental gains in dignity can be as predictive as incremental gains in income, age, or other commonly used health predictors. We fully realize that this does not resolve the issue of whether dignity in fact leads to or causes better health. For instance, we recognize that mental or physical health problems might profoundly shape dignity in their own right, as in the case of feelings of worthlessness leading to lower dignity scores, or serious health problems that lead to foregone autonomy due to disability or incapacitation.

However, we also take multiple strategies to shore up the concern of reverse causality in our cross-sectional approach. First, we establish dignity's association with determinants of health, such as discrimination, resources, social groups, and stress, as well as with health itself. We reason that if dignity associates strongly with precursors of health and with health itself, then it is likely to matter for generating health or well-being, at least in some capacity. Second, we conduct instrumental variable analyses in which we estimate a bidirectional relationship, and we find much stronger support for dignity influencing health rather than vice versa. Third, we reason that if health influenced dignity but not the other way around, then healthier or more advantaged social groups would generally show weaker relationships between dignity and health. Generally, we find this not to be true. Fourth, we reserve the possibility that disability can still compromise dignity. Fifth, we interpret stigma more broadly to include socially minoritized groups, for whom disadvantage was present before any health problems.

# 6

# Dignity as an Efficient Indicator of Social and Moral Integration

How much dignity do Americans perceive in their lives? Table 6.1 shows what we found when we looked at the distributions of the subjective dignity responses in the 2017 and 2021 Gallup surveys.

From 2021 to 2017, we see that negative responses—indicating greater indignity—have increased in their frequencies. Individuals are less likely to agree that they have dignity and are more likely to believe that they do not have it. In Table 6.1, we show in bold the response categories for which "dignity threat" is present: that is, a denial of the dignity of one's life, being treated with dignity, or the ability to control one's dignity.

In the remaining chapters, we take two key approaches to treating these responses, following the last chapter's methodological overview. First, we combine the three items into a subjective dignity scale, and we utilize these scale scores to help understand people's overall sense of dignity that they experience. As we will show, these levels of dignity relate to individual health and well-being as well as to a variety of social, psychological, and economic resources within individual lives and across social groups in society.

Second, we focus on whether individuals are experiencing any dignity threat, and we treat this perceived threat as a particularly salient concern for public health.

Figure 6.1 provides a snapshot of how scale scores and the prevalence of dignity threat changed from 2017 to 2021. We see that the percentage of the Gallup sample reporting any dignity threat rose from 14.1% to 21.5%, amounting to an increase of over 50%. If we expand our definition of indignity to include any neutrality or disagreement on at least one of the three dignity items, these proportions increase to 19.8% and 28.7%, representing about a 45% increase (not shown in Figure 6.1).

As we noted in Chapter 5, we also use multiple indicators of subjective dignity to make a three-item scale. In 2017, the average or mean dignity

*The Science of Dignity*. Steven Hitlin and Matthew A. Andersson, Oxford University Press.
© Oxford University Press 2023. DOI: 10.1093/oso/9780197743867.003.0007

**Table 6.1** Changes in Dignity Responses from 2017 to 2021

|  | Strongly Agree | Agree | Neutral | Disagree | Strongly Disagree |
|---|---|---|---|---|---|
| "I feel that my life lacks dignity." | | | | | |
| 2021 | 5.6% | 7.5% | 2.8% | 36.4% | 47.8% |
| 2017 | 1.5% | 5.7% | 2.3% | 32.2% | 58.5% |

|  | Strongly Agree | Agree | Neutral | Disagree | Strongly Disagree |
|---|---|---|---|---|---|
| "People generally treat me with dignity." | | | | | |
| 2021 | 27.6% | 61.8% | 2.6% | 5.8% | 2.2% |
| 2017 | 34.3% | 58.8% | 1.6% | 4.3% | 1.1% |

|  | Strongly Agree | Agree | Neutral | Disagree | Strongly Disagree |
|---|---|---|---|---|---|
| "I determine my own dignity." | | | | | |
| 2021 | 33.7% | 54.0% | 6.0% | 3.7% | 2.7% |
| 2017 | 40.7% | 49.6% | 4.7% | 2.7% | 2.2% |

*Note:* Percentages within years may not sum exactly to 100.0, due to cell rounding.

## Gallup 2017 Values and Beliefs of the American Public Survey

*Any* Threat to Dignity (Based on All Items):
### 14.1% of National Sample

Subjective Dignity Scale (Normed to 0-1, Based on Three Dignity Survey Items):
Mean = 0.601, Standard Deviation = 0.295 (n = 1468 responses)

## Gallup 2021 Values and Beliefs of the American Public Survey

*Any* Threat to Dignity (Based on All Dignity Survey Items):
### 21.5% of National Sample  (↑ 52.5 % from 2017)

Subjective Dignity Scale (Normed to 0-1, Based on Three Dignity Survey Items):
Mean = 0.529, Standard Deviation = 0.303 (n = 1241 responses)

**Figure 6.1** Dignity Threat and Average Dignity Levels in America from 2017 to 2021

score, once normed to a scale of 0 to 1, was 0.601, with a standard deviation of 0.295. In 2021, the average score was about 15% lower, coming in at 0.529.

We can also look at how Americans are distributed across rough levels of overall dignity (Table 6.2). While the encouraging news from these findings is that most Americans have at least moderate levels of dignity, many Americans do not, and these cases of indignity merit closer examination just as much as the lives within which dignity seems to be abundantly present. Periodically throughout the remainder of this book, we refer to individual dignity items. However, to allow us to speak of "subjective dignity" as an overarching concept, we focus mainly on how individuals scored on the three-item scale ranging from 0 to 1.

As we discussed in Chapter 5, this dignity distribution is similar in form to that of self-rated health at any given time for the U.S. population. Most people feel fine, but those who do not represent significant shifts in social circumstances that deeply affect their sense of well-being, worth, and connection, captured by asking them about their sense of dignity. How do we know dignity is related to, but not simply, a replacement for some of these other concepts? We detail this for the rest of this chapter.

Table 6.2  Changes in Dignity Responses from 2017 to 2021, by Level. Subjective Dignity Scores Across the Pandemic

| Subjective Dignity (Scale Score: 0 to 1) | n/% of Gallup Respondents in 2017 | n/% of Gallup Respondents in 2021 |
|---|---|---|
| Dignity Threat Likely: 0–0.25 (Disagree with Survey Items) | 187 (12.8%) | 233 (18.7%) |
| Threat Possible: 0.25–0.50 (Neutral with Items) | 357 (24.5%) | 369 (29.7%) |
| Threat Unlikely: 0.50–0.75 (Neutral / Agree with Items) | 451 (30.9%) | 337 (27.1%) |
| No Dignity Threat: 0.75–1.00 (Agree with Items) | 464 (31.8%) | 304 (24.5%) |
| Total | 1,459 (100.0%) | 1,243 (100.0%) |
| Average Dignity Level (Std. Deviation) | 0.601 (0.295) | 0.529 (0.303) |

## Starting with a Synonym: Are Dignity and Respect the Same?

We start here with an empirical examination of respect, which often is treated as a synonym of dignity. Of course, scholars such as Donna Hicks have passionately argued that dignity and respect are hardly the same thing: dignity rests in a set of social practices oriented toward humanizing someone as a person, while respect is narrower—that is, it resides in a set of gestures displaying deference toward the social statuses held by individuals, often more focused on a particular situation. This said, Figure 6.2 shows how dignity and respect relate, according to Gallup survey data collected in 2017 and again in 2021.

Looking at these graphs, we see that dignity clearly relates to respect. For instance, individuals are roughly *five times* more likely to "feel disrespected in general" when their levels of dignity are low, compared to higher dignity levels. Taking a domain-specific approach to respect, we see that individuals with higher levels of dignity do indeed feel more respected by their employers

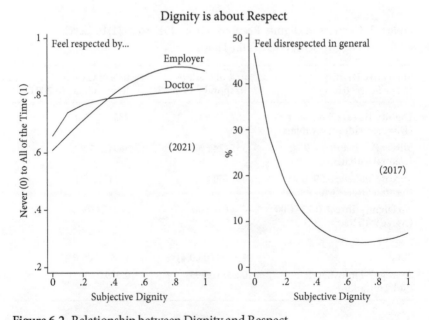

**Figure 6.2** Relationship between Dignity and Respect

*Note:* Gallup respondents were asked whether they feel respected by their ww or doctor (0 = never, 1 = all of the time) and whether they feel disrespected in general.

and their health care providers, which were the two available domain-specific respect items in the 2021 Gallup Values and Beliefs of the American Public dataset. *Just as important, we take away the empirical observation that dignity and respect are not interchangeable.* For instance, barring very low levels of dignity, people are unlikely to feel disrespected in general.

## Dignity Is Weakly Linked to Particular Moral Codes

After respect, individuals often associate dignity with some form of morality. Is dignity tied to specific moral ways of being? If so, then there might be little sense in proceeding to use it for the American population. Here, we see that dignity only is weakly related to perceived accountability to others ("I am accountable to others for how I carry out my responsibilities") and a perceived need to repair any harm done to others ("When I have hurt someone, I try to repair the harm I have caused"), both of which were survey items on the 2021 Gallup survey with a response format focused on agreement versus disagreement (Table 6.3).

Table 6.3   Dignity and General Moral Principles. Subjective Dignity and Its Relation to Generalized Moral Principles

| Subjective Dignity (Scale Score) | % Who Agree They Feel Accountable to Others | % Who Agree They Try to Repair Harm Done to Others |
| --- | --- | --- |
| Dignity Threat Likely: 0–0.25 (Disagree with Survey Items) | 67.1% | 79.4% |
| Threat Possible: 0.25–0.50 (Neutral with Items) | 73.1% | 79.9% |
| Threat Unlikely: 0.50–0.75 (Neutral/Agree with Items) | 75.5% | 84.9% |
| No Dignity Threat: 0.75–1.00 (Agree with Items) | 81.3% | 91.7% |

While accountability and making amends do become more common as dignity increases, even with the lowest levels of dignity we see fairly high levels of agreement. Put another way, dignity seems to be far more than

Table 6.4 Dignity and Specific Moral Beliefs. Subjective Dignity and Its Relation to "Doing the Right Thing"

| Subjective Dignity (Scale Score) | % Expressive Individualist | % Utilitarian Individualist | % Relation/ Authority Oriented | % God Oriented |
|---|---|---|---|---|
| Dignity Threat Likely: 0–0.25 (Disagree with Survey Items) | 24.5% | 12.0% | 29.4% | 34.1% |
| Threat Possible: 0.25–0.50 (Neutral with Items) | 16.8% | 10.1% | 38.1% | 35.0% |
| Threat Unlikely: 0.50–0.75 (Neutral/Agree with Items) | 21.2% | 7.2% | 39.0% | 32.7% |
| No Dignity Threat: 0.75–1.00 (Agree with Items) | 15.7% | 7.2% | 37.9% | 39.2% |

subscription to a general ethic of social responsibility, and such subscription may not even be necessary for the experience of dignity in many situations. There is more variation in people's responses to our dignity items than on these moral orientations.

In Table 6.4, each column corresponds to a perceived source of moral or ethical guidance in response to the question "If you were unsure of what was right or wrong in a particular situation, which of the following best describes how you would decide what to do? (*Please mark only one box.*) Would you: do what would make you feel happy (coded as expressive individualist), do what would help you get ahead (utilitarian individualist), follow the advice of an authority or person you respect (relational/authority orientation), or do what you think God or scripture tells you is right (theistic)?"[1]

Here, we see that individualistic tendencies decrease from low to high levels of dignity, while authority- or God-oriented responses tend increase with dignity. For instance, expressive individualism becomes 36% less common, while a relational or authority orientation becomes 29% more common. This could speak to the more social character of dignity. At the same time, given moral pluralism within the United States, we might expect dignity to be largely independent of any specific justifications for conduct,

---

[1] These categories are modeled after Christian Smith's modification of a question used by Hunter (2000); see Vaisey 2009, 1691. They represent possible orientations as to how people feel they should behave morally.

and that also is consistent with what we see here, since diverse moral codes are present at each dignity level.

Taking the preceding tables together, it would be a mistake to walk away thinking that dignity has little to do with morality. But if dignity is not strictly about a general sense of accountability to others—which is quite common, at least in terms of how people perceive themselves to be—and if it does not strictly inhere in concrete orientations toward God, authority, or one's own individual success, then where can it be found? Instead, perhaps, dignity is to be found more in the *process* of living within society. We consider this possibility moving forward, in terms of dignity's relationships with discrimination, mastery, mattering, meaning, resources, and life stress.

## Perceived Discrimination

Lamont and colleagues (2016) have suggested that perceived discrimination is one of the most consistent routes to indignity. Perceived discrimination, at its root, involves a perception of unfair treatment or being held to a differing, arbitrary standard (Major, Dovidio, and Link 2018; Roscigno, Yavorsky, and Quadlin 2021; Williams 2018). Higher rates of perceived discrimination among minoritized social groups, and robust associations between perceived discrimination and physical—even cardiovascular—health, attest to the structuring of society in ways that create greater harmful stress for minoritized social groups (e.g., Carr and Namkung 2021; Fan, Qian, and Jin 2021; Grollman 2012; Major, Dovidio, and Link 2018).

Based on items available to us within the Gallup survey, one approach to measuring perceived discrimination involves asking individuals whether they think they need to work harder than others to get ahead or at least get noticed for their good work (e.g., Waters and Kasinitz 2010). Table 6.5 breaks down subjective dignity levels based on how often people think this happens within their own lives ("work harder than others to be noticed").

Subjective dignity differences by perceived discrimination are noticeable, more so than what we just saw for differing moral codes. Moving from "never" to "most or all of the time," we see a 33% decrease in dignity levels. Meanwhile, these differences are not as strong as what we saw earlier with feeling disrespected in general, but they are comparable in size for what we saw for specific forms of disrespect such as those linked to one's doctor or employer.

Table 6.5  Dignity and Perceived Discrimination. Dignity
Suffers in the Presence of Perceived Discrimination

| Measure of Perceived Discrimination "How often do you feel like you have to work harder than others to be noticed?" | Average Level of Subjective Dignity |
| --- | --- |
| Never | 0.645 |
| Hardly Ever | 0.601 |
| Some of Time | 0.509 |
| Most or All of Time | 0.432 |

## Closer to the Heart of Dignity: Examining the Three Ms of Mastery, Mattering, and Meaning

Drawing on what we have been piecing together in the earlier chapters, leading scholars and philosophers of dignity suggest that it might be found in more basic human needs.

What are these more basic underpinnings of dignity? Although we reasonably cannot get to the bottom of every philosophical or sociological account of dignity offered, we suggest here that many of these accounts can be articulated in terms of three Ms: **mastery, mattering,** and **meaning in life.** In psychology, organismic approaches to flourishing emphasize autonomy, competence, and relatedness as essential to mental well-being (Deci and Ryan 2000), all of which seem to have deep conceptual alliances with dignity. Similarly, approaches in economics and development studies emphasize how mental or physical well-being stems from freedoms and opportunities present in life above and beyond basic material conditions (Hojman and Miranda 2018; Sen 2000).

First, a sense of autonomy or self-determination seems to be essential. A Kantian perspective views a human life—more precisely, a human mind—as one capable of conscious deliberation and free will. We sociologically modified this Kantian take, in terms of a socially shaped degree of perceived autonomy. While it is difficult to capture a perception of free will in a philosophical sense, decades of psychological research have used perceptions of control or **mastery over life** to tap whether individuals feel that they can create meaningful change or solve problems around them (e.g., Hitlin and

Long 2009; Mirowsky and Ross 2007). If individuals feel fundamentally powerless amid life's struggles, in that their earnest efforts seem to amount to little or nothing, then they also might experience less dignity.

Second, some form of respect or recognition from others seems essential to most theoretical and practical writings on dignity across the centuries. Following this same thread, we began by examining respect in its own right. Now, we transition to a broader consideration of **mattering** to others: beyond feeling respected or disrespected by others, do you also feel that others pay attention to you and make you feel important in some capacity?

Third, though less mentioned, is a notion of purpose or **meaning in life**. While perhaps not necessarily essential to dignity, a sense of meaning seems to tap into adequate social integration, in terms of valued life projects or principles. Because these social involvements can change, one's sense of meaning might falter. One's dignity could potentially falter in response to a deficit in life meaning, perhaps if one does not have a strong sense of control or community to fall back on.

So do these "three Ms"—as proposed, definitional underpinnings of dignity—in fact relate to whether individuals see dignity present within their own lives? Just as important, are any of them so strongly related with dignity that we might argue they are functionally interchangeable or effectively synonymous?

Consider the graphs shown in Figure 6.3, which are based on flexible curve forms to allow uneven or nonlinear relationships whenever shown by the data. The gray lines within each graph depict a relationship for a particular demographic group: men, women, white, Black, Hispanic, less than four-year college education, college education or higher, age less than fifty-five, and age fifty-five or greater. The thick, black line shown within each graph depicts the average trend across all of these demographic groups. We do not label the specific gray lines because they generally uphold and contribute to the average, black line.

Across these graphs, we see that mastery, mattering, and meaning show similarly strong relationships to subjective dignity scale scores, and that these trends have a similar shape across the demographic groups examined.

Dignity clearly is related to all three Ms: higher levels of dignity are found as each of the three Ms increase. Yet, dignity is not interchangeable for any of the three Ms: even for someone who is relatively high in a sense of mastery or mattering, dignity is only predicted to be above average, not maxed out, for example. Likewise at the bottom: for those with lower senses of mastery,

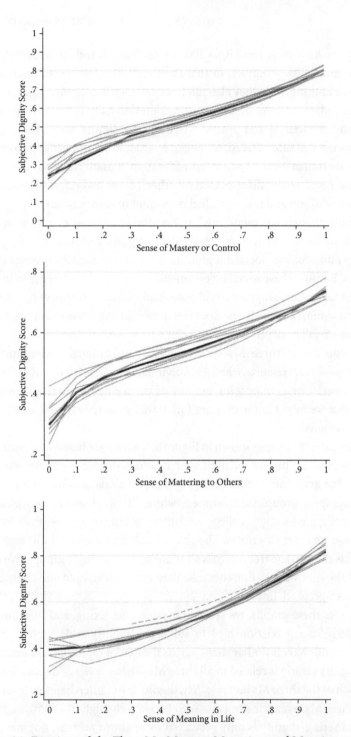

**Figure 6.3** Dignity and the Three Ms: Mastery, Mattering, and Meaning

*Note:* Overall fit for entire Gallup sample shown by thick, black line. Gray lines represent fit lines for demographic subgroups. Dashed line is partially depicted due to inconsistent fit from 0 to 0.3.

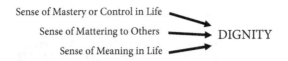

TOGETHER, THESE BIG 3 RESOURCES OVERLAP <u>30%</u> WITH DIGNITY
(<u>70%</u> OF DIGNITY OCCURS BASED ON OTHER LIFE FACTORS)

**Figure 6.4** Dignity and the Three Ms: Summarizing Their Overlap

meaning, or mattering, dignity levels are predicted to be below average to middling, hardly zeroed out. *While dignity significantly correlates with each of these three definitional underpinnings, the relationships are not one to one, supporting the conceptual distinctiveness of dignity.* Taken together, these resources explain about a third of overall dignity levels—which is quite impressive given the numerous inputs to dignity (Figure 6.4).

In Figure 6.4, the calculation of 30% total overlap with dignity—almost one-third—is based on a squared correlation metric known in the social sciences as $R^2$ or "variance explained." In other words, about one-third of the variability in people's dignity scores is accounted for by these three key resource levels. The take-home is that dignity captures these three Ms, as well as many of the other properties we have discussed. If you want specificity in your population analyses, perhaps you need to pick your term; if you want an efficient indicator of individual experiences of social processes, subjective dignity seems to operate quite well.

## Focusing on Economic and Material Disadvantage

If we take away anything from a human rights perspective on dignity, it is that dignity suffers or is compromised under life conditions of social or economic harm or disadvantage. A further test of whether perceptions of dignity align with human rights approaches in a fundamental way would be to examine economic and material disadvantage. While we take a closer look at conditions of disadvantage and indignity in Chapters 8 and 9, we offer a first illustration in Table 6.6.

This table is broken out by survey year and by economic quintile. Economic quintile is determined by a composite of education, income, paid work, and overall economic standing in society. While dignity declines across this time

Table 6.6 Dignity by Economic Background, 2017 to 2021

|  | Subjective Dignity (2017) | Subjective Dignity (2021) | % Change (2017 to 2021) |
|---|---|---|---|
| **U.S. Economic Quintile** | | | |
| 1 (lowest 20%) | 0.545 | 0.403 | −26.0 |
| 2 | 0.590 | 0.533 | −9.7 |
| 3 | 0.619 | 0.549 | −11.3 |
| 4 | 0.668 | 0.613 | −8.2 |
| 5 (highest 20%) | 0.705 | 0.643 | −8.7 |

period were observed across the board—for all economic groups—the disadvantaged were hit over twice as hard, declining by 26% relative to the more modest declines for other economic segments. We turn to specific, resource- and stress-based reasons behind this general trend in the coming chapters.

## Summary: Do We Have an Efficient Indicator?

In view of the evidence presented here, we take a moment to revisit the motivating question of this chapter: do we have an efficient indicator of moral and social integration in society? To be able to answer in the affirmative, we would need to be able to show not only that dignity relates to its presumed definitional underpinnings but also that it is not simply interchangeable with these underpinnings.

Dignity carries considerable promise as an efficient indicator, based on the evidence gathered from the 2017 and 2021 Gallup Values and Beliefs of the American Public surveys. Tantamount to the way self-rated health reflects underlying diseases, symptoms, or illnesses, dignity captures some of the presumed, more objective underpinnings of a well-integrated life in society. And, just as for self-rated health, dignity is not interchangeable with these underpinnings. Because it is not interchangeable, it holds the potential to add something to scientific studies: to explain health and well-being in an efficient, encompassing way that other social indicators might overlook. We turn to health and well-being in the next chapter.

# 7

# Is a Dignified Life a Healthier Life?

Based on the research we reviewed in the first chapters of the book, it might seem like any association between dignity and health would be almost self-evident. How could there not be one? After all, proposed definitional pillars of dignity, such as autonomy, lack of violence, humiliation or abuse, social integration and relationships, and viewing oneself favorably or with some esteem, all have established social scientific links to mental or physical health.

So, is dignity's importance for health naturally evident from all this research on similar concepts? Perhaps. But the link is hardly automatic. Given ample disagreements about what dignity is or what it might look like, it may be too imprecise or wide-ranging to mean anything deep enough to most individuals to correlate with bodily or mental health.

*Here, we offer health measures as a way of establishing subjective dignity as not just a moral, cultural, or rhetorical term—but rather as a potential public health concern.* What is at stake in an examination of dignity and health is whether dignity is understood to be sufficiently personal, and not just an element of public culture that people talk or equivocate about (Lizardo 2017; Swidler 1986, 2001). For a time, "happiness" studies were quite popular in English-speaking countries; we might suggest that another indicator of social relations would have been to focus on dignity, rather than happiness, as it gets closer to capturing the range of social and moral properties and experiences we have discussed thus far.

## The Shape of the Association: Trajectory- and Group-Based Approaches to Dignity and General Health

We begin here by thinking about health in terms of a trajectory: that is, one's past health, one's current health, and one's future health. Is your health getting better or worse? We implement an eleven-point self-rated health item used in the Gallup survey that allows to compare across these temporal

*The Science of Dignity.* Steven Hitlin and Matthew A. Andersson, Oxford University Press.
© Oxford University Press 2023. DOI: 10.1093/oso/9780197743867.003.0008

Table 7.1  Dignity and Past, Present, and Future General Self-Rated Health

| Subjective Dignity | Past Health | Current Self-Rated Health (0 to 10) | Future/Anticipated Health |
|---|---|---|---|
| 0 to 0.2 (lowest) | 7.6 | 6.5 | 6.1 |
| 0.2 to 0.4 | 7.8 | 7.1 | 6.7 |
| 0.4 to 0.6 | 8.0 | 7.3 | 7.1 |
| 0.6 to 0.8 | 8.2 | 7.4 | 7.2 |
| 0.8 to 1.0 (highest) | 8.5 | 7.9 | 7.8 |

perspectives. Recalling the last chapter, we focused on the example of a five-category, classic self-rated health measure. Here, we use eleven categories because this is a version of self-rated health called a self-anchoring measure, also commonly used among epidemiologists and economists. It reads, "On a scale from zero to 10, where zero represents the worst possible health for you and 10 represents the best possible health for you, please rate your health at the following points in time: your current health, your health 10 years ago, and your expected health 10 years in the future." The results are shown in Table 7.1.

Across the past, present, and future, greater dignity is associated with greater health. Average responses to these self-rated health items fall between about 6 and 8.5, and people generally expect worse health looking ten years into the future due to anticipated, natural declines in wellness due to aging processes. By a similar logic of bodily aging, self-rated past health shows the highest levels. In published research, we find that the association between subjective dignity and self-rated health holds across numerous demographic groups determined by age, race, ethnicity, education, income, political ideology, and labor force status (Andersson and Hitlin 2022).

How large is the association between dignity and health? Generally, dignity's association with self-rated health and depressive symptoms is quite similar in strength to the association we see for income. The other lines drawn are for mastery, mattering, and meaning in life—our three Ms from the last chapter—and for perceived economic status, the gold standard subjective social status measure. Overall, dignity performs around the same magnitude as all these comparisons, although mastery or control is a bit stronger in terms of how big of a span of self-rated health or depressive symptoms it covers (Figure 7.1).

Comparing Associations of Key Resources with Physical/Mental Health

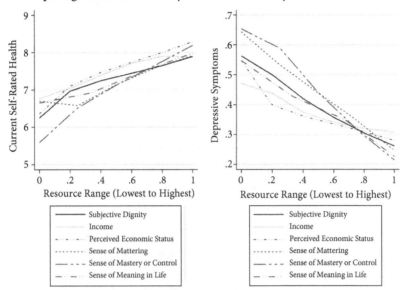

**Figure 7.1** Associations between Health and Dignity, Compared to Other Key Associations

## Dignity as a Public Health Concern: How Widespread Are the Links to Health Indicators?

Across the 2017 and 2021 Gallup survey data, we incorporated a variety of health and well-being indicators. With few exceptions, we found significant associations of indignity with specific health indicators. The graph in Figure 7.2, also shown in the book's Introduction, presents the percentage increases in health or well-being problems associated with reporting indignity. Again, indignity is defined in terms of disagreeing that one has dignity on at least one of the dignity items on our survey.

Overall, the results are striking. People who report potential dignity threats demonstrate *nine* distinct health or well-being ailments relative to respondents who show no dignity threat. Against this baseline category, elevations in percentages range from about a 35% increase in physical inactivity to about a 270% increase in not feeling happy. (A 100% increase constitutes doubling—and a 200% increase is tripling—of the rate observed among those without dignity threat.) Most percentage increases are somewhere between 50% and 125% or so, quite significant from a practical and

DIGNITY as a Public Health Issue

Depressed ↑ 130 % (vs. no threat)
Unhappy ↑ 268 %
Angry ↑ 66 %
Difficulty Sleeping ↑ 35 %
Feels Left Out ↑ 95 %
Current Smoker ↑ 76 %
Physical Inactivity ↑ 35 %
Bored ↑ 51 %
Fair/Poor Health ↑ 136 %

*whenever any dignity threat is present*
*(21.5% of United States in 2021)*

**Figure 7.2**  Health Risks Associated with Lower Levels of Dignity

statistical standpoint. Smoking, difficulty sleeping, feeling left out, feeling bored or angry, feeling depressed, and reporting fair or poor general health are all substantially more likely among those under dignity threat.

Indignity is associated most strongly with feeling depressed or not happy or being in fair or poor self-rated health. Indignity is not the cause of these behaviors, necessarily, but an indicator that some people's life circumstances are far from ideal, and that perception is strongly related to a range of health issues.

## Which Direction? Investigating the Link between Dignity and Health from Both Sides

Why does dignity show such a strong link to health?

Well, one possibility is that impaired dignity degenerates physical well-being over time, through elevated stress response, worsened health behaviors such as smoking or poor diet, lowered optimism or sense of control, or other, resource-based pathways that we will unpack in more depth in the next chapter.

Another possibility, however, is that health problems themselves lead to a sense of indignity, perhaps due to improper health care or how our society treats people who live with physical or mental disabilities.

Both pathways are worth considering. To disentangle them properly, we would need longitudinal data where we tracked the same people's dignity levels over time as well as their changing health information. Without that,

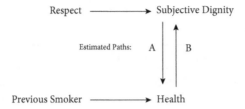

**Figure 7.3** Using Instrumental Variables to Estimate Bidirectional Associations between Dignity and Health

however, we still can offer a meaningful test of both possibilities using the available data.

Using the 2017 Gallup data, we conducted an instrumental variable analysis. In the social sciences, instrumental variable models can be used to try to figure out the prevailing directionality of a potentially bidirectional relationship. Does dignity associate with better health, or is it the other way around?

To devise the instrumental variable analysis, we can take advantage of two facts: (1) whether people perceive themselves to be respected is linked strongly to, but not interchangeable with, whether they perceive dignity in their lives, and (2) childhood family adversity and being a previous smoker are predictive of current health levels (Ferraro, Schafer, and Wilkinson 2016) and do not significantly relate to dignity after accounting for health. These earlier experiences sort people into different levels of dignity and thus help us gain better insight into dignity's relationship to health.

Across two different ways of assessing self-rated health, and across two different statistical techniques for estimating the magnitudes of bidirectional effects,[1] we find that the evidence is more consistent with dignity causing better health rather than vice versa (Figure 7.3 and Table 7.2).

As reported above, the estimated relationship between dignity and health is approximately 1.6 units on the self-anchoring measure shown earlier in this chapter. In other words, from the lowest to the highest levels of dignity, we would expect a health gain of about 1.6 points on this measure.

However, this statistical analysis does not isolate the unique, stigmatizing impact that disability or physical or mental health limitations can have in our society. As we clearly argued in Chapter 4, ableism is a pillar of American

---

[1] We implement full-information maximum likelihood (FIML) and two-stage least squares (2SLS) (Paxton et al. 2011).

Table 7.2 Results from Instrumental Variable Procedure for Dignity and Health

**Self-Rated Health (0 = Poor to 1 = Excellent)**

| Instrumental Variable | Previous Smoker | | Lived with Two Parents Growing Up | |
|---|---|---|---|---|
| Model Estimator | FIML | 2SLS | FIML | 2SLS |
| Path | | | | |
| A (Dignity --> Health) | 0.203*** | 0.208*** | 0.198*** | 0.199*** |
| B (Health --> Dignity) | 0.053 | 0.106 | −0.014 | −0.024 |

**Current Self-Rated Health (0 = Worst Possible to 10 = Best Possible)**

| Instrumental Variable | Previous Smoker | | Lived with Two Parents Growing Up | |
|---|---|---|---|---|
| Model Estimator | FIML | 2SLS | FIML | 2SLS |
| Path | | | | |
| A (Dignity --> Health) | 1.615*** | 1.706*** | 1.614*** | 1.644*** |
| B (Health --> Dignity) | −0.009 | 0.016 | −0.009 | −0.003 |

FIML = Full Information Maximum Likelihood Estimation; 2SLS = Two-Stage Least Squares Estimation; *** denotes statistical significance at $p < .001$ (two-tailed test)

capitalism. We take up this concern more directly in Chapter 9, where we analyze dignity differences by health limitation status.

## Control It All Away: Is It Really Dignity Improving Health, or Is It the Conditions Surrounding Dignity?

The social conditions creating dignity are multifaceted and interwoven. Given this, what would it mean to say that dignity leads to better life outcomes?

We are using mail- or web-based surveys to record numeric levels of dignity and health. People's levels of dignity exist prior to our survey, and we are not sure what caused them. In fact, the social and personal inputs leading to their dignity are probably far too complex to measure perfectly.

In social life, we are led into certain situations by virtue of the resources we do or do not have or the pressures we do or do not face—or by our values or our personalities. Life presents obstacles and we pressure ourselves to do certain things. As a paraphrased saying goes, nothing in real life is left to chance.

These external pressures are confounding forces when it comes to observational research. In the words of Yale medical sociologist and physician Nicholas Christakis, they "confound" our ability to know what is really happening. Is it the conditions surrounding and creating dignity or is it dignity itself that is behind any differences in health that we see across people?

Close readers of the first part of the book probably are shrugging at this point. We are too, to some extent. After all, dignity emerges from a set of social, economic, and psychological conditions, and it is not separable from these conditions. To put it simply, dignity *is* these conditions—inheres in these conditions—and it is the *perception* and *experience* of these conditions.

So, then, is it a fool's errand to try to "eliminate" confounders and thereby identify dignity's "real" effect? This is a complicated question, one that is equal parts philosophical and mathematical. However, because we are social scientists, we can follow the conventions of our field. We can do what most observational, quantitative researchers do, and use control variables to make our findings more convincing. However, one risk we run by accounting for confounding conditions using control variables is what might be termed an *underestimation* of the true effect that dignity has. By controlling away the conditions surrounding dignity, we might be statistically washing out the phenomenon itself, in other words.

Yet, at the same time, robustness of any observed associations between dignity and health to a comprehensive accounting of surrounding conditions could provide added confidence that our findings are not merely the result of having higher income, or being married, or being white, or being a Democrat or a Republican, and we believe this sort of demographic confounding is useful to address.

Thus, we undertook a multivariable, controlled analysis of the estimated associations between subjective dignity and depressive symptoms and subjective dignity and self-rated health. This lets us have added confidence that dignity's value holds across diverse social backgrounds and is not specific to any of these backgrounds. We show our findings in Table 7.3.

In this confounding-corrected analysis, we obtain the estimated associations between dignity and depressive symptoms and self-rated health, net of differences in education, income, marital status, working part or full time, urban or rural residence, political ideology, sex, race or ethnicity, and age. Paying attention to the "Subjective Dignity" row, we can compare that magnitude to what we saw depicted in the earlier graphs. For instance, the estimated effect of dignity (what statisticians would call "b" or beta) on

Table 7.3 Adjusted Associations between Dignity and
Health (Including Control Variables)

|  | Depression, b (95% CI) |
| --- | --- |
| Subjective Dignity | −0.242 (−0.298, −0.186) |
|  | Self-Rated Health, b (95% CI) |
| Subjective Dignity | 0.164 (0.107, 0.223) |

depressive symptoms is −0.242. This means that, across the entire range of dignity from 0 to 1, we would expect depressive symptoms to drop by −0.242 units. Because we had also scaled depression to a range of 0 to 1, this turns out to be quite a large estimated effect, on par with a difference of tens of thousands of dollars in income. Similarly, for self-rated health, we see a difference of 0.164. Here, self-rated health has been rescaled to range from 0 to 1 as well. This again is a substantial association. The numbers you see in parentheses represent the 95% confidence interval for these estimated effects; in other words, we are 95% confident that the "true" effect lies between the two parenthetical numbers, at least based on the analysis we have conducted.

## A Preview of What's to Come: How Does Dignity Relate to Health under Extreme Life Stress?

When it comes to associations between dignity and health, can we use these more complicated, multivariable models to show that dignity is linked to health above and beyond the "three Ms" that researchers have used for a long time before incorporating any notion of "dignity" into their analysis of health and well-being? For someone whose life lacks a sense of control, who feels they do not matter to others, or who feels at a loss for their life's meaning, can dignity still be a last resort or a stopgap for buffering their well-being? To put it colloquially, if someone "at least" has their dignity, can their health be buffered in turn?

Before we show the results, we want to offer two caveats that for many readers would nullify the importance of these results. First, these three Ms, according to many scholars at least, could be viewed as necessary or at least useful conditions for obtaining a sense of dignity. A second caveat, no

**Table 7.4** Adjusted Association between Dignity and
Depressive Symptoms (Including Control Variables and
the Three Ms of Mastery, Meaning, and Mattering)

|  | Depression, b (95% CI) |
| --- | --- |
| Subjective Dignity | −0.061 (−0.109, −0.014) |

smaller than the first, is that the three Ms could be experienced and occur
right around the same time that dignity is measured.

The estimated net effect is shown in Table 7.4.

As you can see, the estimated effect has diminished by about 75%, down to
−0.061 from the −0.242 we showed earlier. However, even under these very
extreme conditions, dignity still is linked to significant differences in depressive symptoms.

For self-rated health, we instead see something remarkable. Dignity
becomes more, not less, protective of self-rated health as the three Ms (here
called "the Big 3") fade away. Dignity really does seem to be a health buffer
for individuals experiencing a lack of mattering, less mastery, and lower
meaning in life. Individuals lower on these important resources—below the
50th percentile—show a positive, stronger association between dignity and
health (Figure 7.4).

For depressive symptoms, we do not find any straightforward interaction
effect. It could be that depressive symptoms are a bit too closely linked to the
phenomenon of dignity for dignity to play a meaningful buffering role.

## Summary and Looking Toward Next Chapters

Subjective dignity—the degree to which individuals think "dignity" is in
place within their own lives—is linked to better mental and physical health.
This association holds across many ways of measuring health and is present
across a variety of segments of the population as well. The shape of the relationship is a generally increasing one—more dignity relates to better health,
level by level.

While one might interpret this widely observed association between dignity and health in terms of favorable bodily health leading to a sense of dignity, this interpretation is not supported. In fact, dignity appears to buffer

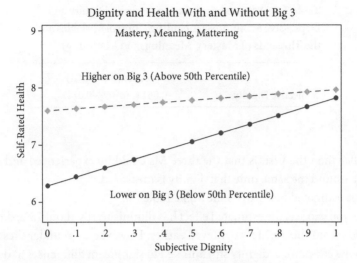

**Figure 7.4** Dignity Shows a Stronger Relationship to Health When Mastery, Meaning, and Mattering Are Lacking

health especially among those who are suffering from a lack of perceived control, meaning, or mattering within their lives, suggesting this subjective perception might serve a unique role in *promoting* favorable health, rather than just reflecting pre-existing differences in health.

Across the next two chapters, we make a closer consideration of resources and adversities to paint a more tangible portrait of how dignity relates to well-being in America. Perceptions of dignity could lead to better health because dignity emerges from pathways involving psychological, social, and economic resources that promote health, a case we begin to build in the next chapter. Also, dignity could be associated with differences in experiencing or reacting to stress, an explanation we unpack in the following chapter.

# 8

# A Resource-Based Framework
# for Analyzing Levels of Dignity

Many Americans perceive indignity in their lives. If dignity is important for staying healthy or maintaining well-being, as we have suggested, then how might one go about obtaining it? By many definitions, dignity indicates how one fits into their social roles, statuses, or networks. How malleable is dignity, given that it measures in large part how others view us?

Suppose that dignity is distributed randomly—like a lottery—or, alternatively, that dignity is a mindset that one chooses. If so, we might expect little to no connection between dignity and the resources characterizing individual lives. However, as we are beginning to see across our analyses, dignity is a product of how societies and individuals relate, and the obstacles and resources that play into that dynamic and potentially difficult relationship. In this chapter, we look at the economic, psychological, and social resources in people's lives, and how those relate to levels of subjective dignity in our lives.

## One Road or Many Roads? Outlining a Resource-Based
## Argument on Social Variation in Dignity

Societal resources are doled out unequally, as we discussed earlier in conjunction with American capitalism and its interlocking systems of inequality. Not everyone gets ahead in life: some of us are in a better position to accumulate resources, and we do not all have the same starting points. We can examine this empirically, using various economic, psychological, and social resources measured across the 2017 and 2021 Gallup surveys (Table 8.1).

**Economic resources** capture one's socioeconomical resources in terms of money, education, availability of work, availability of food, and availability of health insurance.

*The Science of Dignity*. Steven Hitlin and Matthew A. Andersson, Oxford University Press.
© Oxford University Press 2023. DOI: 10.1093/oso/9780197743867.003.0009

Table 8.1 Overview of the Dignity Resource Model

| Economic Resources | Psychological Resources | Social Resources |
| --- | --- | --- |
| Has Health Insurance | **Sense of Mastery or Control** | **Sense of Mattering to Others** |
| Perceived Standing in Society | | |
| Lack of Financial Strain | Sense of Resilience | Feeling Close to Family |
| Food Secure | **Sense of Meaning in Life** | Feeling Close to Friends |
| Income | | Feeling Close to Neighbors |
| | Optimistic about 10-Year Goals | Feeling Close to Coworkers |
| | Overall Religiosity or Spirituality | Trust in Others |
| **Educational Level** | | Church Attendance |
| Works Full Time | | Religious Friend Group |
| | | Have Significant Other |
| | | Close to Online Community |

Educational level is examined separately as a cornerstone of economic, psychological, and social resources. Senses of mastery, meaning, and mattering show the strongest individual contributions to
predicting dignity levels.

**Psychological resources** refer to perceptions we have about the world that
affect our behavior: whether we feel in control, resilient, like our lives are
meaningful, and optimistic about what our future might hold, and possibly
whether we approach the world in a religious or spiritual way. Importantly,
decades of sociological research have shown that these psychological resources are not measures of idiosyncratic mindsets: they profoundly reflect history, power, and status, and social circumstance more generally
(Andersson 2012; Elder 1994; Frye 2012; Emirbayer and Mische 1998; Hitlin
and Johnson 2015; Mirowsky and Ross 2007).

**Social resources** are about the web of relationships we cultivate and in
which we find ourselves: whether we are connected to people who see us as
mattering; whether we feel closeness to significant others and our different
communities, organizations, and work groups; whether our connections inspire an overall sense of trust; whether we are partnered; and whether we
connect meaningfully with those we know in the digital sphere.

In some ways, resources beget resources, leading the socially rich to become socially richer (e.g., DiPrete and Eirich 2006; Ferraro 2018; Ferraro,
Shippee, and Schafer 2009; Ferraro, Schafer, and Wilkinson 2016; Jackson
2015; Link and Phelan 1995), much like how financial processes operate. For

instance, having health insurance could increase one's sense of control over life, and being food secure could make one more optimistic about one's future. Meanwhile, education increases income and often enhances trust in society; working full time generates income and could also generate some meaning in life; and work, education, or religiosity could be associated with meeting a significant other. There are many more examples: the bottom line is that resources tend to reinforce one another both within and across domains or categories.

In both 2017 and 2021, if we define having an economic, psychological, or social resource as having a resource that is dichotomous in nature (e.g., health insurance, having a significant other) or as being around or above moderate levels of resources that have multiple levels, we can generate an overall resource count for each respondent in our survey. In doing so, we connect dignity to resource count in general, and we see that a higher overall count of resources is linked to greater dignity levels (Table 8.2).

Table 8.2  Dignity Levels across Overall Resource Counts, 2017 and 2021

|  | Subjective Dignity (2017) | Std. Dev. | Subjective Dignity (2021) | Std. Dev. |
|---|---|---|---|---|
| Count of Resources | | | | |
| ≤2 | 0.186 | 0.172 | 0.237 | 0.232 |
| 3 | 0.396 | 0.327 | 0.325 | 0.271 |
| 4 | 0.326 | 0.321 | 0.344 | 0.272 |
| 5 | 0.410 | 0.290 | 0.447 | 0.305 |
| 6 | 0.480 | 0.237 | 0.460 | 0.268 |
| 7 | 0.475 | 0.254 | 0.480 | 0.287 |
| 8 | 0.586 | 0.257 | 0.565 | 0.290 |
| 9 | 0.600 | 0.303 | 0.546 | 0.264 |
| 10 | 0.607 | 0.276 | 0.586 | 0.273 |
| 11 | 0.669 | 0.271 | 0.659 | 0.281 |
| 12 | 0.716 | 0.244 | 0.693 | 0.270 |
| 13 | 0.754 | 0.219 | 0.726 | 0.290 |
| 14+ | 0.813 | 0.234 | 0.724 | 0.242 |
| Total Range in Dignity | 0.627 (0.813–0.186) | | 0.487 (0.724–0.237) | |

## For Dignity, Having More Resources Generally Is Better

There clearly is a strong relationship between dignity and overall resource count. Across the entire resource count, ranging from less than or equal to two resources all the way up to fourteen or more resources, one sees a difference in dignity of over 0.6 in 2017 and about 0.5 in 2021. This is a very large range: in fact, it spans the difference between indignity and perceiving great dignity in one's life.

At the same time, the relationship between resource count and dignity level is a bit uneven, since there are marked jumps in dignity across some specific resources. Also, for each count of resources from less than or equal to two to fourteen-plus, there is much variation in dignity, as denoted by the standard deviation (Std. Dev.) at that rank. What might explain this wide variation in scores, even among those with the same count of resources? At least two key explanations for this variation will be addressed next.[1] First, specific resources show differing degrees of overlap with dignity. That is, resources vary quite a bit in terms of how much they correlate with dignity. We turn to this issue next. Second, resources connect to dignity differently across different segments of the population. To uncover these group-specific trends, we estimate resource overlaps separately by demographic group.

## When It Comes to Dignity, What Resources Matter Most?

In Chapter 6, we provided an overview of the trends connecting dignity to the three Ms of mastery, mattering, and meaning in life. We saw that all three of these associations were quite strong, although none of them came close to being interchangeable with dignity, in terms of how much they overlap. Here, then, we take a moment to show how all the ranges of additional psychological, economic, and social resources stack up when it comes to their overlap with measured levels of subjective dignity.

As mentioned in the last chapter, we make use of the squared correlation ($R^2$) coefficient, which is defined as the square of the correlation coefficient, $r$. Again, we can think of $R^2$ as being similar to a Venn diagram: as $R^2$

---

[1] Of course, other explanations for rank-specific dignity variation exist, such as differences in the most prevalent resource combinations at and across given resource counts.

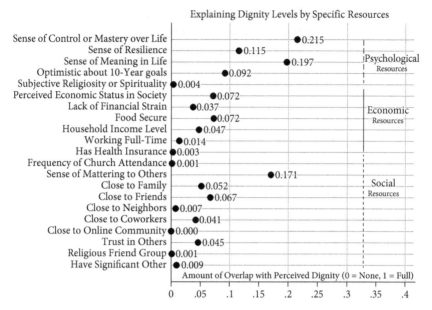

**Figure 8.1** Overlap between Dignity and Specific Psychological, Economic, and Social Resources

approaches 1, there is increasing overlap between the circle of dignity and the circle of a particular resource. Figure 8.1 shows the degree of observed overlap with dignity.

As this overlap plot shows, dignity is not a story of any one resource, but rather is more like a story of how multiple resources combine to shape a life and its dignity. As we can see here, mastery, meaning, and mattering remain the strongest predictors of dignity, measured in terms of how much they overlap with dignity. These "three Ms" have overlaps near or greater than 0.2. All the other resources show some overlap, but not nearly as much. Other resources with substantial overlap include resilience and optimism; perceived status in society; lack of difficulty paying bills; food security; income; closeness to friends; and so on. Generally, we would expect that some resources might factor more strongly into feelings of dignity at certain times than at other times, depending on the situation in which one finds oneself.

But do different groups in society think of dignity in the same way? What about group-specific differences in the applicability of this resource model?

**Table 8.3** Dignity Ranges Linked to Resource Count, by Demographic Group and Survey Year

|  | Total Range in Dignity (from 2 to 14+ Resources) | |
| --- | --- | --- |
|  | 2017 | 2021 |
| Overall | 0.627 | 0.487 |
| Men | 0.620 | 0.590 |
| Women | 0.659 | 0.471 |
| White | 0.639 | 0.435 |
| Black | 0.403 | 0.568 |
| Hispanic | 0.785 | 0.451 |
| <College Degree | 0.643 | 0.590 |
| College Degree+ | 0.771 | 0.549 |
| Age <35 | 0.633 | 0.556 |
| Age 35–55 | 0.684 | 0.310 |
| Age >55 | 0.532 | 0.471 |
| Single | 0.748 | 0.559 |
| Married | 0.628 | 0.331 |

Now, we ask how well a resource-based perspective explains the dignity levels that we see *across different demographic groups*. As before, we start with a summary of dignity range and resource count (see Table 8.3). Overall, dignity ranges widely according to resource count as we discussed earlier: by 0.627 in 2017 and by 0.487 in 2021. While the dignity range attached to a resource model is similar for men and women in 2017, it is noticeably greater for men in 2021. Meanwhile, there is substantial racial and ethnic variation in dignity range across both survey years. Variations by educational level, age, and marital status are apparent as well.

Because overall resource count does not reveal which resources might matter more to the dignity of particular social groups, we produced a table of overlap ($R^2$) statistics defined by resource and group. Table 8.4 reveals the specific dignity-resource dynamics by sex, race, and education, averaging across both survey years.

While we will not offer a detailed discussion of all of these findings, it does present a striking illustration of how resource dynamics are similar but also

**Table 8.4** Particular Overlaps between Resources and Dignity, by Demographic Group

| Resource Types/Facets | Overall | Men | Women | White | Black | Hispanic | <College | College+ |
|---|---|---|---|---|---|---|---|---|
| | Overlap with Dignity (0 = None; 1 = Complete) | | | | | | | |
| **Psychological Resources** | | | | | | | | |
| Sense of Mastery over Life | 0.22 | 0.24 | 0.20 | 0.21 | 0.17 | 0.23 | 0.22 | 0.18 |
| Sense of Resilience | 0.12 | 0.11 | 0.13 | 0.11 | 0.05 | 0.17 | 0.09 | 0.15 |
| Sense of Meaning in Life | 0.20 | 0.23 | 0.19 | 0.22 | 0.05 | 0.25 | 0.20 | 0.21 |
| Optimistic (10-Year Goals) | 0.09 | 0.11 | 0.07 | 0.09 | 0.04 | 0.15 | 0.09 | 0.08 |
| Religiosity or Spirituality | 0.00 | 0.00 | 0.00 | 0.00 | 0.03 | 0.01 | 0.00 | 0.01 |
| **Economic Resources** | | | | | | | | |
| Perceived Standing in Society | 0.07 | 0.08 | 0.07 | 0.10 | 0.06 | 0.04 | 0.07 | 0.03 |
| Lack of Financial Strain | 0.04 | 0.04 | 0.05 | 0.05 | 0.01 | 0.05 | 0.04 | 0.01 |
| Food Secure | 0.07 | 0.07 | 0.09 | 0.07 | 0.01 | 0.14 | 0.07 | 0.03 |
| Household Income | 0.05 | 0.05 | 0.05 | 0.07 | 0.01 | 0.04 | 0.03 | 0.04 |
| Works Full Time | 0.01 | 0.03 | 0.00 | 0.02 | 0.00 | 0.00 | 0.01 | 0.00 |
| Has Health Insurance | 0.00 | 0.00 | 0.01 | 0.00 | 0.00 | 0.02 | 0.00 | 0.00 |
| **Social Resources** | | | | | | | | |
| Frequency of Church Attendance | 0.00 | 0.00 | 0.00 | 0.00 | 0.02 | 0.01 | 0.00 | 0.01 |
| Sense of Mattering to Others | 0.17 | 0.20 | 0.16 | 0.18 | 0.08 | 0.21 | 0.17 | 0.17 |
| Feeling Close to Family | 0.05 | 0.05 | 0.06 | 0.06 | 0.00 | 0.11 | 0.05 | 0.06 |
| Feeling Close to Friends | 0.07 | 0.05 | 0.09 | 0.08 | 0.02 | 0.08 | 0.08 | 0.04 |
| Feeling Close to Neighbors | 0.01 | 0.01 | 0.01 | 0.01 | 0.01 | 0.01 | 0.00 | 0.03 |
| Feeling Close to Coworkers | 0.04 | 0.02 | 0.07 | 0.03 | 0.02 | 0.10 | 0.03 | 0.04 |
| Close to Online Community | 0.00 | 0.00 | 0.00 | 0.00 | 0.03 | 0.02 | 0.00 | 0.00 |
| Trust in Others | 0.05 | 0.03 | 0.07 | 0.06 | 0.00 | 0.08 | 0.04 | 0.04 |
| Religious Friend Group | 0.00 | 0.00 | 0.00 | 0.00 | 0.00 | 0.00 | 0.00 | 0.00 |
| Have Significant Other | 0.01 | 0.02 | 0.00 | 0.01 | 0.00 | 0.02 | 0.01 | 0.01 |

different across social groups. Resources represent many, but certainly not all, ways of increasing a sense of dignity. Social groups carry different social and cultural histories that will need to inform future research into the measurement of dignity resources. An absence of resources or different meanings attached to resources could reflect a backdrop of stress or adversity, which we turn to in the next chapter.

## Education: A Cornerstone Connecting Dignity and Health in America

Modern societies are centrally structured around educational systems that shape adult economic and psychological resources. Economists and sociologists of many persuasions have come around to the fact that early, compulsory, and postsecondary education is a key foundation of many if not most resources during adulthood, and that educational success and persistence are profoundly structured by family socioeconomic status growing up (Calarco 2014, 2018; Heckman and Krueger 2003; Heckman 2006; Mirowsky and Ross 2003). In other words, while it is not the sole determinant of later-life resources, education shapes most of the resource trajectories that we identified in the last section. Especially important is whether one obtains higher levels of education past high school, or one's final educational level (what sociologists refer to as educational attainment).

This is not to say that families or communities are irrelevant for generating one's stock of resources throughout life. Many of us have our parents or communities to thank, at least in part, for how well or decently our lives turned out. Yet, the point remains: families and communities are structured in ways that are designed to enable (or at least not limit) the educational process from being productive. If a community cannot produce enough high school graduates, that community generally also suffers from several social and economic obstacles in the continuation of its safe or prosperous existence.

Just as the economists Anne Case and Angus Deaton (2021) have recently termed an educational divide in American "deaths of despair," we outline how this general educational process might operate in the production of many resources across the life course that promote and protect health and well-being while also increasing life expectancy.

<pre>
                       Resources
College Degree   →    Economic     →  Subjective
   Attainment    →  Psychological  →   Dignity
                 →     Social       →
</pre>

**Figure 8.2** Differences in Resources Lead to Greater Dignity among College Graduates

## Higher Education as a Cornerstone of Economic, Psychological, and Social Resources during Adulthood

While no two college experiences are created equal in terms of institution, curriculum, mentoring, or prestige, it still is useful to speak in general terms about how postsecondary education plays into diverse resource trajectories within American society. Postsecondary schooling includes a variety of two- and four-year credentials, although four-year credentials tend to carry higher lifetime economic, psychological, and social resource premiums than two-year credentials, at least on average (Zajacova and Lawrence 2018, 2021). This said, we consider this general set of radiating pathways (Figure 8.2).

Within this diagram, we have placed "college degree" in a position where it leads to differences in economic, psychological, and social resources during adulthood, all of which in turn play into one's overall, subjective sense of dignity. In other words, this is a resource-based argument for how dignity operates in society, with education given special emphasis, based on over a half century of empirical social science research.

College graduates have higher levels of most—all but three, in fact—of the psychological, economic, and social resources we listed earlier (Table 8.5).

## Breaking Down the College Resource Premium

Not only are the resource differences linked to a college degree quite large, but also they are wide-ranging, spanning a variety of psychological, economic, and social resources. College graduates are better off in terms of their senses of control, resilience, meaning, and optimism; health insurance, perceived status in society, lack of difficulty paying bills (i.e., financial strain), food security, income, and probability of landing full-time work; feeling like they matter to others; feeling close to their families, friends, and communities; being embedded in trusting social networks; and having larger

**Table 8.5** Divides in Psychological, Economic, and Social Resources, by College Degree Status

| Resource Types/Facets | % with Resource, <College Degree | % with Resource, College Degree+ | College Premium |
|---|---|---|---|
| **Psychological Resources** | | | |
| Sense of Mastery over Life | 56 | 64 | +14% |
| Sense of Resilience | 66 | 70 | +5% |
| Sense of Meaning in Life | 47 | 57 | +21% |
| Optimistic (10-Year Goals) | 78 | 90 | +15% |
| Religiosity or Spirituality | 78 | 71 | −10% |
| **Economic Resources** | | | |
| Perceived Standing in Society | 32 | 69 | +117% |
| Lack of Financial Strain | 43 | 62 | +42% |
| Food Secure | 62 | 86 | +39% |
| Income (About or Above Average) | 41 | 73 | +81% |
| Works Full Time | 36 | 53 | +45% |
| Has Health Insurance | 90 | 97 | +7% |
| **Social Resources** | | | |
| Frequent Church Attendance | 52 | 48 | −8% |
| Sense of Mattering to Others | 48 | 53 | +10% |
| Feeling Close to Family | 63 | 66 | +4% |
| Feeling Close to Friends | 63 | 67 | +6% |
| Feeling Close to Neighbors | 59 | 56 | −5% |
| Feeling Close to Coworkers | 47 | 58 | +23% |
| Feeling Close to Online Community | 19 | 22 | +17% |
| Trust in Others | 67 | 81 | +21% |
| Religious Friend Group | 46 | 55 | +20% |
| Have Significant Other | 54 | 62 | +14% |

networks inside and outside of organizations, in addition to the well-known fact that college graduates are more likely to be stably partnered or married than nongraduates (Hout 2012; Mirowsky and Ross 2003).

Putting all these resources together, it is no wonder that college graduates feel—and are—better off in American society. Put another way, American society is structured in ways that clearly reward college graduates. One might even say, echoing the language of the social epidemiologist Bruce

Link, that college degrees are veritable cornerstones ("fundamental causes") of health-promoting resources. In fact, as Michèle Lamont has observed, the concentration of economic and social rewards among college-educated professionals in our society is part of the reason our society has become so starkly fragmented in terms of politics and in terms of life prospects and chances (Lamont 2019). All of this, Lamont contends, is paramount to understanding the growing dignity divide within American society.

Thus, it seems that education truly is a cornerstone of many adult resources, in terms of its foundational role in shaping higher valuation and return on these resources. Generally, in America, individuals complete schooling before they go on to start a full-time career. Although plenty of individuals work while in college, these jobs typically are not the same jobs that they hold after graduation. College graduation generally leads to other job opportunities, which are more stable and higher paying and thus can lead to growing economic, psychological, and social resources.

We are fully aware that full-time work of any kind is its own source of stress, as it takes a toll through limited time for community involvement and through work-family conflict, for example. We take up the issue of varying experiences of overwork more directly in Chapter 9.

Before we learn more about how these resource pathways function under stressful circumstances, what else can we discover about the association between college and dignity?

## Staying Connected: A Quick Application to Pandemic Dignity and the Dark Side of Social Networking

Since we are heading toward a discussion of stress and the pandemic in the next chapter, we offer a quick application here as a way of rethinking the recent American upheavals as affecting these social resources. While we have already seen that the social resources of closeness to family and friends and embeddedness in a trusting community each show associations with subjective dignity, it is unclear how this translates to a situation where in-person interaction is entirely removed or dramatically reduced, as we have seen during much of the Covid-19 pandemic.

As a starting investigation, we might draw a distinction between online and in-person closeness and ask how each type of closeness—and how particular combinations of in-person and digital interaction—is linked to dignity

(Figure 8.3). Keeping in mind the sociological phenomenon of copresence (Goffman 1967), which involves entrainment between individuals due to co-ordination of thoughts and nonverbal and verbal signals (Campos-Castillo and Hitlin 2013), we might expect that digital interaction could be an effec-tive substitute for in-person interaction, at least in terms of establishing a sense of "being" with someone. Whether digital interaction has an equally potent link to dignity, however, remains to be seen.

One thing we learn from Figure 8.3 is that feeling close to family and friends is more important to dignity than whether one took up greater online socializing with these close ties during the pandemic. However, if one man-aged to maintain a sense of closeness while also interacting online, this espe-cially increased dignity, as shown by the topmost bar (0.645). Moving online in its own right offers some contribution to dignity, but not nearly as much when felt closeness is lacking (0.475).

This all might make online socializing seem like a purely positive thing as far as dignity is concerned. However, we know all too well from instances of online disagreement, altercation, or harassment and from cases of cyberbul-lying and social media "canceling" of influencers that what happens online has the potential to harm the people involved. If one has an uneasy or nega-tive experience with online interactions or social media, this appears to chip

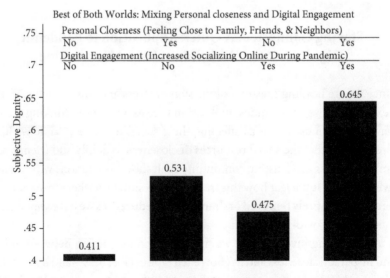

Figure 8.3  Dignity and Mixed-Mode Social Integration

Dignity in Detachment: Emotional Distance from Online Life

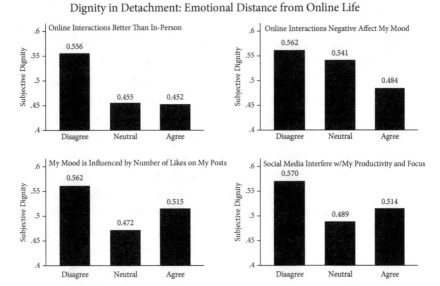

**Figure 8.4**  Greater Dignity Linked to Keeping Distance from Online Life

away at dignity just as much as whether one goes online at all or as much as differences in real-life emotional closeness to family and friends (Figure 8.4).

Following Figure 8.4, we see that a strong preference for online interaction and a feeling of being deeply influenced by social media (events or likes) is linked to unfavorable levels of dignity relative to greater "detachment," where we think preferring real-life interaction and managing one's emotions and time spent on social media. But is it really this simple? It still seems possible that if one witnesses a troubling notification or an offensive post, a single event could become a watershed moment in one's evolving experience of dignity with the digital sphere. This is an avenue for future research.

## Summary

Levels of subjective dignity vary substantially across individuals in society. Given this fact, we need to be able to account systematically for why individuals experience their lives with varying levels of dignity. While some of this variation certainly is based in individual interpretations of what dignity means, we nonetheless still see striking patterns of how societal inequality structures these dignity perceptions. In other words, individual variation in experiences of dignity is quite socially predictable based on the levels of resources held by individuals. Resources are doled out unequally among individuals, according to the macro structures of capitalism discussed earlier in the book.

A resource-based perspective, developed in this chapter, draws on a variety of psychological, economic, and social resources to reveal a key set of explanations for why some individuals experience more dignity than others. American life is structured in ways that place more resources into the hands of some individuals over others, and this can help us understand why some individuals report greater dignity. Indeed, dignity itself is linked to resources: the more resources, the more dignity one perceives in one's life, although some resources are more tightly linked to dignity perceptions than others. In view of the digitalization of many real-life encounters, we might profitably think of reconceptualizing some social resources in terms of online interaction dynamics rather than strictly in-person quantifications.

Meanwhile, one important limitation of a resource-based perspective to consider is that cultural meaning-making processes, social processes of adversity or trauma or discrimination, personal biographies and interpretations of dignity, and other factors beyond a resource model can also matter. However, our streamlined focus on resources, broadly understood, allows us to better situate dignity within the web of some resources that tend to matter in our society. Beyond the resources we have, it is important to consider the stressful conditions under which these resources are put to the test or rendered ineffective due to individual or collective trauma, an issue we take up in our next chapter, which deals with dignity and adversity.

A cornerstone connecting dignity, health, and resources among adults is college education. Americans are obtaining college degrees now more than ever, and those without college degrees are being left behind in ways that hold real consequences for leading a life perceived as dignified. These dignity perceptions rest in how American society is structured to disproportionately reward college graduates—while leaving nongraduates behind psychologically, socially, and economically. Qualitative work over the past two decades has argued this, and we offer perhaps the first national survey-based support for this contention.

In fact, a dignity-based accounting of resource levels might help us make better sense of what Case and Deaton have called "deaths of despair" among white Americans. Quite possibly, as Case and Deaton and Michèle Lamont have suggested, it is not just a relative lack of opportunity and resources but also the associated social stigma and degradation of self-inherent in dignity that reinforces these material disadvantages, in turn leading to elevated, lethal substance use. While we cannot yet offer a conclusive contribution to understanding this larger social issue, we fully agree with Lamont's assessment that dignity and inequality are deeply connected, and those who are left behind in resources also are left behind in terms of their experienced dignity and, relatedly, their health. To help build out our evidence base for how dignity, resources, and health connect, we next turn to the differing levels of stress that individuals encounter.

# 9

# Inequality and Stress

## Charting Dignity during Social Adversity

A resource-based perspective, outlined in the last chapter, gives us a textured appreciation for how inequality shapes dignity, based on where people are in their resource trajectories. Inequality, understood abstractly, translates into measurable resources that, in turn, foster dignity to a greater or lesser extent. However, the story of social inequality is more than just one of resource differences. It is also one of differences in stress, stigma, and exclusion (Case and Deaton 2021; Lamont et al. 2016; Lamont 2019).

Indeed, when it comes to our analysis of dignity, we have only begun to scratch the surface of inequality. For instance, we have not begun to seriously consider levels of dignity due to inequalities by race, sex, age, disability, or other characteristics that carry categorical or group-based implications for life chances within American capitalism.

Meanwhile, American society has endured recent, further stressors related to the unfolding Covid-19 pandemic. Of course, these Covid-related stressors have been distributed unequally by sex, race, age, and other demographic characteristics. Amid conditions of collective stress, differing social groups experience levels of stress that are markedly varied, due to how these groups are positioned in society in terms of their historic and cultural levels of prestige, status, wealth, and power.

Therefore, we develop in this chapter a stress-based perspective to complement a resource-based perspective. Stress, broadly understood, tends to erode individual resources (Pearlin and Bierman 2013) while also offering a separate, distinct set of explanations for patterns in dignity levels. Resources focus more on positive or favorable aspects of life, while stress revolves more around obstacles and endurance necessitated by the structural conditions of our society.

In understanding group differences in dignity levels between 2017 and 2021, it helps to show percentage decreases in their own right (Table 9.1).

*The Science of Dignity.* Steven Hitlin and Matthew A. Andersson, Oxford University Press.
© Oxford University Press 2023. DOI: 10.1093/oso/9780197743867.003.0010

**Table 9.1** Dignity Declines and Levels from 2017 to 2021, by Demographic Group

| Demographic Group | % Change (2017 to 2021) | Subjective Dignity (2017) | Subjective Dignity (2021) |
|---|---|---|---|
| College Degree+ | −8.6 | 0.653 | 0.596 |
| Black | −17.0 | 0.651 | 0.570 |
| Hispanic | −14.1 | 0.637 | 0.565 |
| Women | −14.7 | 0.631 | 0.565 |
| Married | −7.6 | 0.617 | 0.547 |
| 25–39 Years | −8.1 | 0.614 | 0.540 |
| 55–69 Years | −11.4 | 0.607 | 0.538 |
| 40–54 Years | −11.5 | 0.603 | 0.538 |
| Overall | −12.0 | 0.601 | 0.534 |
| White | −11.4 | 0.594 | 0.529 |
| 70+ Years | −18.5 | 0.592 | 0.526 |
| <College Degree | −16.5 | 0.583 | 0.522 |
| Asian | −3.0 | 0.583 | 0.487 |
| Men | −9.0 | 0.574 | 0.483 |
| American Indian | −13.1 | 0.557 | 0.483 |
| Single | −14.4 | 0.552 | 0.472 |
| <25 Years | −20.1 | 0.530 | 0.423 |

Before laying out a stress-based perspective on dignity levels, we start by providing an overview of general dignity levels by demographic group (see Andersson and Hitlin 2022 for more details on these group-based differences). Because the pandemic enfolds a considerable depth and diversity of social stress, we break out dignity separately by pre- and during-pandemic levels as well. In line with the college cornerstone argument presented in the last chapter, we see the highest levels of dignity, demographically speaking, among college graduates (0.653 in 2017 and 0.596 in 2021). Whatever happened during this time period, having a college degree remained one of dignity's biggest buffers.

Returning to the college-related inequalities for just a moment, we now can see that the college-dignity divide is usefully understood not just in terms of absolute levels of dignity by year but also in terms of the precipitous drop in dignity we see among nongraduates from 2017 to 2021 (16.5%) relative to the drop seen among graduates, which was considerably milder (8.6%).

Women experienced a greater decrease in dignity than did men; racial minorities saw a larger decrease than Whites; and young (younger than twenty-five years) and older (seventy-plus years) showed some of the largest increases. Perhaps quite surprisingly given the increased prevalence of violence toward Asian Americans during the pandemic, Asian Americans showed the smallest observed decrease against all groups (just 3.0%). Across all groups (i.e., "overall"), the average observed dignity decrease was 12.0%.

How do we begin to make sense of these changes? Because social perceptions and objective life conditions both matter to dignity, it might be most useful to view these decreases as reflecting a combination of shifting cultural and group-specific standards as well as shifting cultural and group-specific resources. For instance, perhaps groups confronting a lack of socioeconomic mobility, or structural discrimination within society, find ways of redefining dignity that refuse to concede to injustice and instead place a greater emphasis on solidarity and community. Despite these attempts to refashion the criteria one uses to judge one's life in a self-protective way, the events between 2017 and 2021 seem to have eroded most people's sense of dignity.

Put another way, redefinition of dignity represents both a political act and a way of reclaiming dignity (e.g., Bourgois 2003; Oeur 2016). Ellis Monk has conceptualized this possibility in terms of linked fate among African Americans (Monk 2020), and Hispanic and Asian communities have resisted hegemonic narratives of dignity based in restrictive approaches to acculturation or citizenship (Van Hook and Glick 2007, 2020). While Native Americans did not suffer the greatest losses of dignity, they started and remained at some of the lowest levels of dignity seen in the United States. Enduring, continued challenges to their lands and communities—beyond restricted access to food, water, and health care—may overwhelm any cognitive or collective efforts to redefine dignity.

In fact, Lamont's cross-national perspective on dignity (Lamont et al. 2016; Lamont 2019) shows how dignity is about far more than social class, job conditions, or educational levels. Religious, racial, and ethnically minoritized groups in societies around the world perform acts of boundary work—drawing moral lines—to distinguish criteria they use to view themselves as worthy from how society might view their group from the outside. If the wider society does not offer the tools for a sense of dignity, groups will create their own to enable their continued sense of moral worth.

Table 9.2  Intersecting Race and Gender to Understand Dignity Levels,
2017 to 2021

|  |  | Subjective Dignity (2017) | Subjective Dignity (2021) | % Change (2017 to 2021) |
|---|---|---|---|---|
| *White* | Men | 0.564 | 0.527 | −6.6% |
|  | Women | 0.625 | 0.523 | −16.3% |
| *Black* | Men | 0.593 | 0.554 | −6.6% |
|  | Women | 0.690 | 0.541 | −21.6% |
| *Hispanic* | Men | 0.629 | 0.520 | −17.3% |
|  | Women | 0.641 | 0.568 | −11.4% |

While some researchers might make "double jeopardy" or "triple jeopardy" predictions, in terms of how combinations of minoritized statuses might be detrimental to health or other outcomes (e.g., Robinson 2016; Yang, Jackson, and Zajicek 2021), the reality for subjective dignity is a bit more complicated (Table 9.2).

We see that a greater loss of dignity among women compared to men is strongest among Blacks and Whites and not present among Hispanics. Keeping in mind the rapidly escalating childcare and domestic responsibilities brought on by the pandemic, and how these responsibilities can obstruct career devotion, one can build a narrative for greater dignity loss among women; once we add the additional dynamic of race, we can recognize that extended kin obligations and pandemic-related economic and health adversity occur more commonly among Blacks than among Whites. This could help us make sense of the relatively precipitous loss of dignity among Black women.

To help build out these group-specific profiles in more detail, we turn now to a fuller accounting of the stressors endured during the pandemic—and of how these stressors each relate to dignity levels. When it comes to thinking about stress and dignity, it helps to begin by thinking about levels of exposure to different stressors across the pandemic (Table 9.3).

Generally, we can understand differences in subjective dignity across the pandemic not just in terms of the psychological, economic, and social resource model introduced in Chapter 8 but also in terms of the stress-based exposures shown in Table 9.3. However, these stressors were endured by some demographic groups in society far more than others.

**Table 9.3**  Declines in Dignity Associated with Major Social Stressors, and Prevalence of Stressor by Demographic Group

| | Associated Decline in Dignity | Estimated Prevalence in U.S., Spring 2021 (%) | Relative Prevalence (1.00× = Equal) | | | |
|---|---|---|---|---|---|---|
| | | | Women vs. Men | Black vs. White | Hispanic vs. White | Sexual/ Gender Minority |
| *Lost Job* | −0.107 | 10.1 | 1.26× | 2.00× | 2.65× | 2.41× |
| *Reduced Work Hours* | −0.058 | 21.2 | 0.99× | 1.52× | 1.92× | 1.56× |
| *Missed Payments* | −0.091 | 7.3 | 1.76× | 3.01× | 2.32× | 1.73× |
| *Pay Cut* | −0.068 | 13.8 | 1.09× | 1.23× | 2.26× | 1.50× |
| *Went Hungry* | −0.200 | 6.1 | 1.35× | 1.57× | 2.77× | 2.30× |
| *Serious Conflict at Home* | −0.157 | 15.4 | 1.74× | 1.31× | 1.36× | 2.28× |
| *Couldn't Afford Health Care* | −0.154 | 16.0 | 1.46× | 0.86× | 1.26× | 2.19× |

As we can see from the table, the well-documented feminization of poverty is evident during the pandemic, in terms of women being more likely than men to have missed house or rent payments and also being more likely to lose a job due to their disproportionate placement in service jobs rather than salaried jobs. Meanwhile, they are more likely than men to go hungry, to report enduring conflict at home, and to not be able to afford needed health care. Looking into racial and ethnic differences, we see that Blacks and Hispanics are more than twice as likely to endure job loss or hunger or missed house or rent payments. Finally, we unpack differences in Covid stress between those who do not and do identify as sexual or gender minorities (SGMs; Hsieh and Shuster 2021). Like women, Blacks, and Hispanics, SGMs show increased prevalence of all manner of serious pandemic stress.

## Returning to Ableism: How Disabled Individuals Fared across the Pandemic

Through the chapter so far, we have covered aspects of structured economic disadvantage, racial, gender, sexual, and parental differences during

Table 9.4  Dignity by Physical Ability Status, 2017 to 2021

| U.S. Adults Aged 35–55 | | Subjective Dignity (2017) | Subjective Dignity (2021) | % Change (2017 to 2021) |
|---|---|---|---|---|
| *Physical Ability Status* | Disabled | 0.582 | 0.456 | −21.6% |
| | Not Disabled | 0.657 | 0.611 | −7.0% |

the pandemic. Now, we take a moment to unpack differences related to physical ability, another axis on which capitalism perpetuates social inequality. Some sense of control seems to be central to dignity, according to the philosophical and sociological explorations we discussed earlier in the book; we might expect a lack of physical capacity to damage one's sense of dignity, something exacerbated by the isolation brought on during the pandemic. Among those Gallup respondents who reported a health problem limiting their daily activities and who are middle-aged adults, we find that the pandemic was more than three times as devastating to subjective dignity (Table 9.4).

To help understand these tolls, we can look to the realms of health, work, economic resources, and social resources, finding that disabled individuals were less advantaged across all these realms (Table 9.5). In short, these adults were likely to have more limited health, work, financial, and network resources, many of which could help to explain their relatively lower levels of dignity. We recognize here that the restriction to ages thirty-five to fifty-five creates a focus on working-age adults who are likely to have family or parental responsibilities.

## Summary

A stress-based perspective complements a resource-based viewpoint on dignity differences in society. Generally, vulnerable or minoritized groups experienced larger decreases in subjective dignity across the pandemic, although there were some exceptions to this trend. These exceptions might be attributable to boundary work that redefines what dignity means or meaning-making processes among these groups promoting solidarity or coping in a way that buffers dignity levels. These possibilities merit exploration by future

**Table 9.5**  Fewer Health, Work, Financial, and Social Resources
for Dignity among Physically Disabled

|  | Any Physical Disability | | Difference (1.00×=Equal) |
|---|---|---|---|
|  | No | Yes |  |
| *Health* | | | |
| *Fair/Poor Health* | 5.9% | 44.9% | 7.61× |
| *Covid Positive* | 17.1% | 29.5% | 1.73× |
| *Work* | | | |
| *Full-Time Work* | 72.0% | 47.2% | 0.53× |
| *Lost Job* | 12.0% | 12.6% | 1.05× |
| *Hours Reduced* | 23.4% | 29.9% | 1.28× |
| *Finances* | | | |
| *Money to Save* | 36.1% | 15.9% | 0.56× |
| *Missed Payments* | 7.4% | 14.8% | 2.00× |
| *Increased Debt* | 25.6% | 42.5% | 1.40× |
| *Went Hungry* | 7.8% | 14.9% | 1.91× |
| *Social Network* | | | |
| *Close to Others* | 65.9% | 61.0% | 0.93× |
| *Social Online* | 63.0% | 52.9% | 0.84× |
| *Covid Death* | 24.5% | 33.0% | 1.35× |
| *Serious Conflict* | 14.6% | 27.0% | 1.85× |

research better equipped to unpack changing viewpoints on dignity itself
and how these relate to coping or to changing forms of stress.

When intersecting race and gender, we found that women's decreases in
dignity were most striking among Black women, whereas men's decreases
were most striking among Hispanic men. More broadly, we understood
stress-related declines in dignity in terms of different Covid-related stressors,
how each of these stressors related to changes in dignity, and finally in terms
of group gaps in the prevalence of stressors. Overall, notable racial, gender,
and sexual minority gaps are present in terms of economically advantaged,
White, male, and straight/cisgender respondents reporting fewer and less diverse forms of stress and thus less dignity loss overall during the pandemic.

Disability carries multiple ramifications for dignity, especially in times
of additional societal hardship. Physically limited respondents lost dignity
at roughly twice the rate as those without a health limitation from 2017 to

2021, and these losses can be understood in part through different health, work, financial, and network experiences. Although we do not specifically track changes in resources among this group, we instead focus on the fact that experiences among disabled individuals in the 2021 survey were strikingly different across these life realms when compared to the experiences of more able-bodied individuals.

While the patterns of stress and dignity uncovered in this chapter are generative, they might provoke many questions related to other population groups represented by different combinations of age, class, race, or gender, part of the movement toward intersectionality across the social sciences. We are hopeful that the general approach taken in this chapter can inspire these future directions of research as the world continues to navigate a new, different, and complex future. Well-documented shifts in societal functioning and distinctions among people with different privileges and resources operate all the way inside the most personal aspects of the person; the pandemic accentuated existing processes.

# 10

## One Polarized Nation

### Dignity across Political Ideologies

In the preceding chapters, we have examined dignity across a variety of demographic and economic groups, in terms of group-specific resources and stress and how they connect to dignity levels. However, we have not touched on politics, which is perhaps one of the brightest and most contentious dividing lines in American public life, not to mention Covid-related health outcomes (Sehgal et al. 2022).[1] Given how Americans organize so much of how they think and believe around their political ideology (Boutyline and Vaisey 2017), politics deserves its own separate examination. How might we proceed to show that dignity carries value across party lines for understanding American levels of health, resources, and stress?

Our approach to this chapter on politics and dignity resembles how we have proceeded in previous chapters. Here, we offer a reinterpretation of several of our previous findings, broken out separately by political orientation. Then, we link a measure of political polarization itself to levels of subjective dignity across all demographic corners of society.

To manage our presentation here, we focus mainly on political ideology. We have two main reasons for this choice: (1) ideological orientation tends to be somewhat more consistent over time than partisan alignment, and (2) ideological orientation organizes a wider variety of specific policy positions and moral or social beliefs, compared to partisanship or voting patterns (Boutyline and Vaisey 2017). As we touch on later in the chapter, Democrat and Republican voting patterns are associated with similar levels of sensed polarization in society.

---

[1] See also "The Changing Political Geography of Covid-19 over the Last Two Years," Pew Research, March 3, 2022; "Trump Counties Have Higher COVID Death Rates," *US News & World Report*, February 3, 2022.

*The Science of Dignity.* Steven Hitlin and Matthew A. Andersson, Oxford University Press.
© Oxford University Press 2023. DOI: 10.1093/oso/9780197743867.003.0011

Table 10.1  Changes in Dignity by Political Ideology, 2017 to 2021

| Political Ideology | Subjective Dignity Score (2017) | Subjective Dignity Score (2021) | % Change (2021 vs. 2017) |
|---|---|---|---|
| Conservative | 0.594 | 0.534 | −10.1% |
| Moderate | 0.590 | 0.535 | −9.3% |
| Liberal | 0.631 | 0.520 | −17.6% |

## Levels of Dignity across the Pandemic: Liberals Lost the Most

Across the pandemic, people from all political ideologies lost some of their subjective dignity, with liberals losing about twice as much as conservatives and moderates (Table 10.1). In 2021, levels of dignity look remarkably similar across ideology, whereas in 2017, liberals report slightly more dignity. Overall, none of these political viewpoints prevented dignity loss across the ensuing years, and one might ask why exactly it is that liberals lost the most.

Based on the resource and stress mechanisms presented in the preceding two chapters, one might suggest that liberals have lower levels of psychological, economic, or social resources relevant to dignity, as well as greater exposure to—as well as perhaps greater attention paid, or credibility given to—the threat of the pandemic. Whether through frontline work, economic hardship, or greater adherence to protective measures, all these explanations for the lower levels of dignity seem plausible, and we evaluate each to the extent possible with our Gallup data later in this chapter.

Before we proceed to examine these different explanations of the disproportionate loss of dignity among liberals, we want to confirm that dignity holds similar, general meanings across ideology, which we do briefly here by revisiting some of the analyses we presented in Chapter 6 concerning the presumed definitional underpinnings of dignity.

## Across Ideological Lines, Dignity Is About Some of The Same Basic Things

First, we see that the trends associating respect to dignity look remarkably similar based on political ideology (Figure 10.1). Respect is fundamental to

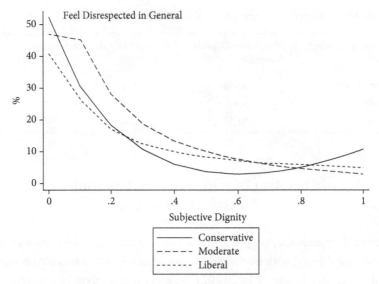

**Figure 10.1** Dignity and General Disrespect, by Political Ideology

how individuals think about dignity. We do, however, see a slightly stronger association among conservatives. Generally, however, individuals who feel a full or complete sense of dignity (around 0.8 to 1.0, the maximum level) are about four to five times less likely to feel disrespected by the individuals around them when compared to those reporting the lowest levels of dignity. In some ways, this is useful to confirm, because if dignity is *not* about respect, then it is not about whether society can or cannot violate dignity, and more about an intrinsic or species-given sense of dignity that cannot be touched by society. So, seeing this general pattern helps cement the interpretation that dignity is about social vulnerability regardless of where one stands.[2]

Likewise, we see similarly potent associations between dignity and health by ideology (Table 10.2). Across ideology, a lack of dignity is most strongly linked to being in fair or poor health or depressed or not happy. Associations with difficulty sleeping, physical inactivity, and anger are relatively similar

---

[2] Of course, how one views respect and the maintenance of it, and how one goes about being respectful, represents a separate set of moral and interactional issues worthy of exploration by further research.

Table 10.2  Dignity as a Public Health Issue, by Political Ideology

| Change in Health or Well-Being Indicator | Conservative | Moderate | Liberal |
|---|---|---|---|
| Depressed | +161.8% | +132.1% | +100.4% |
| Fair/Poor Health | +140.5% | +146.3% | +140.4% |
| Not Happy | +354.4% | +190.6% | +285.9% |
| Physical Inactivity | +25.8% | +27.9% | +16.02% |
| Current Smoker | +68.0% | +33.8% | +123.3% |
| Difficulty Sleeping | +41.7% | +35.1% | +26.6% |
| Bored | +81.1% | +54.0% | +23.0% |
| Angry | +82.1% | +50.9% | +61.4% |
| Feels Left Out | +137.4% | +103.4% | +56.6% |

*Note.* +100% represents *twice* the rate of a health or well-being impairment among those experiencing dignity threat (when compared to those without any dignity threat).

Table 10.3  Dignity Range Linked to Resource Count, by Political Ideology and Survey Year

| | Total Range in Dignity (from 2 to 14+ Resources) | |
|---|---|---|
| | 2017 | 2021 |
| Overall | 0.627 | 0.487 |
| Conservative | 0.428 | 0.718 |
| Moderate | 0.659 | 0.421 |
| Liberal | 0.596 | 0.530 |

by ideology, while feeling bored, feeling left out, and currently smoking are more distinct by ideology.

Having established that dignity relates to health across political divides, we turn back to the resource model. We see some differences in dignity range across resource count by political background in 2017 and in 2021 as well. However, the resource model still receives considerable support regardless (Table 10.3).

We also offer an overview of squared-correlation ($R^2$) overlap by political background. Moderates diverge noticeably from conservatives and

**Table 10.4** Overlaps between Dignity and Specific Resources, by Political Ideology

| Resource Types/Facets | Conservative | Moderate | Liberal |
|---|---|---|---|
| | Overlap with Dignity (0 = None; 1 = Complete) | | |
| **Psychological Resources** | | | |
| Sense of Mastery over Life | 0.182 | 0.244 | 0.238 |
| Sense of Resilience | 0.064 | 0.166 | 0.125 |
| Sense of Meaning in Life | 0.172 | 0.349 | 0.130 |
| Optimistic (10-Year Goals) | 0.064 | 0.128 | 0.079 |
| Religiosity or Spirituality | 0.013 | 0.004 | 0.001 |
| **Economic Resources** | | | |
| Perceived Standing in Society | 0.093 | 0.070 | 0.043 |
| Lack of Financial Strain | 0.023 | 0.051 | 0.038 |
| Food Secure | 0.039 | 0.091 | 0.076 |
| Income (About or Above Average) | 0.039 | 0.053 | 0.045 |
| Works Full Time | 0.006 | 0.020 | 0.016 |
| Has Health Insurance | 0.000 | 0.005 | 0.003 |
| **Social Resources** | | | |
| Frequent Church Attendance | 0.000 | 0.001 | 0.014 |
| Sense of Mattering to Others | 0.180 | 0.192 | 0.145 |
| Feeling Close to Family | 0.060 | 0.041 | 0.073 |
| Feeling Close to Friends | 0.092 | 0.055 | 0.052 |
| Feeling Close to Neighbors | 0.008 | 0.006 | 0.012 |
| Feeling Close to Coworkers | 0.025 | 0.040 | 0.050 |
| Feeling Close to Online Community | 0.026 | 0.020 | 0.000 |
| Trust in Others | 0.038 | 0.037 | 0.055 |
| Religious Friend Group | 0.021 | 0.003 | 0.000 |
| Have Significant Other | 0.005 | 0.009 | 0.017 |

liberals in how dignity relates to particular resources, and conservatives and liberals differ somewhat from each other as well (Table 10.4).

Meanwhile, these general and ideology-specific patterns speak to an overarching reality for dignity: psychological, economic, and social resources linked to a college degree in America matter for dignity regardless of where one stands ideologically.

"Please indicate whether you feel that people in the following groups

threaten the unity of American society."

□ Not a threat   □ Somewhat a threat   □ Very much a threat

- Latinos
- Conservative Christians
- Democrats
- Whites
- Atheists
- Native Americans
- Republicans
- Muslims
- Blacks
- Buddhists
- Asian Americans
- Immigrants

**Figure 10.2**  Gallup Survey Question about Group-Related Polarization in America

## Where Does This Leave Us? Revisiting How Polarization Relates to Dignity Levels in America

If individuals across ideological backgrounds see that dignity is about respect and experience dignity according to these resources and stresses within their lives, then how should we be thinking about the perceived threats affecting all of us, regardless of how we perceive social reality?

We have already addressed pandemic-related threats in terms of liberals' greater declines in dignity relative to those seen among conservatives or moderates. But there is more to the story, especially considering how political polarization affects all of us. How, then, might we measure how polarization is affecting dignity in America? To do this, we can take advantage of a variety of items in the 2021 Gallup survey that asked the question shown in Figure 10.2.

We can think of polarization not just in terms of a general sense of threat pervading society but also in terms of the specific groups that an individual perceives as threatening. Of course, depending on ideology, the groups identified as threatening will differ. Because subjective dignity is tethered in a sense of social resources and integration into society, perceptions of social threat may be enough to chip away at an individual's sense of dignity (Figure 10.3).

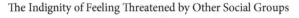

The Indignity of Feeling Threatened by Other Social Groups

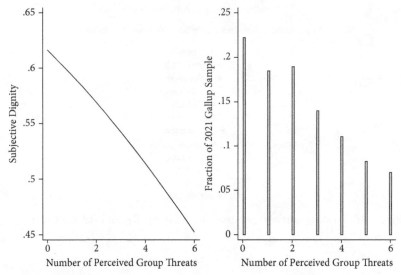

**Figure 10.3** Dignity Declines with Increasing Number of Perceived Group Threats

Those who perceive threats coming from several groups in society are far less likely to feel dignified. Also, about half of the Gallup sample feels threatened by three or more distinct groups in society. Not only is this the case, but also it is the case that individuals across a variety of demographic backgrounds all perceive roughly the same level of threat in society, regardless of which groups seem threatening to which individuals (Figure 10.4).

All groups of survey respondents generally have a mean threat level hovering around 2.0. However, these threat levels are a bit more variable once one focuses on "high threat level," or the percentage of a survey response group perceiving four or more threats, displayed in the right panel of Figure 10.3. Still, though, roughly a quarter of each group falls into this category.

One might maintain that any perceived group threat is a potential threat to social order, in some way. This brings us back to what we said earlier regarding the maintenance of dignity through personal social worlds. In Chapter 3, we set out the argument that dignity is about experiences of care, however one defines or approaches care in one's life, and that it is about the practicalities of routine, relationships, and how we are transformed by and

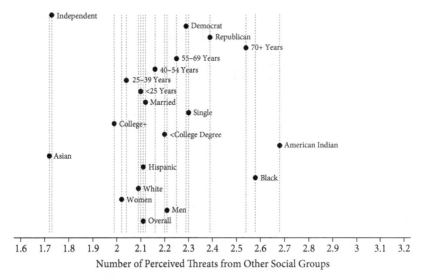

**Figure 10.4** Number of Perceived Group Threats, by Demographic Group

relate to others who are important to us as we live our lives. Perhaps, in view of the above results, we should be thinking of these personal social networks as refuges from a larger social fabric.

Dignity is linked to health and well-being regardless of ideological background, and resources matter for dignity, regardless. What is striking from earlier chapters is that most people say that they have some degree of dignity in their lives. However, since polarization is a looming perception of threat beyond one's local social world, we might gain even more dignity across society by realizing how much of it we might gain by restoring a larger sense of order, one that draws new bridges beyond our socially distanced personal networks.

We begin to sort through some possibilities for larger forms of cultural and moral integration for America in the concluding chapter.

# Conclusion

## Moving Forward

### Dignity's Role in Collective Consensus and Social Inspiration

By letting people determine what dignity means for them, we learn more about how health and well-being are distributed in society. As an efficient indicator of social circumstances, dignity is not left to chance: it is patterned profoundly by resources and stressors in our society, and by group-specific social situations in America. Dignity's absence, as we show, presents a major public health issue. We employ dignity as an indicator of social circumstances, while holding open the possibility that seeking to achieve dignity drives some forms of social action.

In line with the psychologist Susan Fiske's (2004) summary of human motivation, when somebody feels they belong, are understood by and trust others, and are in some control of their fates, and can present to the world a positive self-image, they generally report greater levels of dignity. Despite the particular social and cultural situations affecting historically and economically vulnerable groups in America, we nonetheless find that dignity's association with numerous facets of health and well-being is not restricted to specific groups. Rather, dignity generally is related to having a purpose, having meaningful relationships, feeling in control of one's life, and having enough resources and respect to live well, which are basic, human concerns that we all face regardless of background.

Across multiple years of national survey data, we find that dignity is anything but a lofty term. It is treated by respondents as a practical, real experience. The subject of centuries of contentious scholarship, we find dignity is neither overly abstract nor "useless." Following our findings, dignity has earned a central place in the lexicons of many philosophers, policymakers, and human rights advocates for good reason.

In line with centuries of definitional pluralism that have obscured what dignity "really means," no single factor on its own can fully explain the wide-ranging variation in dignity that we see in our analyses of Gallup survey data. Instead, dignity seems to be a product of numerous psychological, social, and economic resources that individuals accumulate over a lifetime. Also, social groups vary significantly in how they think about dignity: that is, how they draw correlations or links among resources, stress, and dignity levels.

Many of these resources are easier to accumulate in America if one is a college graduate, due to profound resource and stress divides linked to obtaining higher education. As Michèle Lamont (2019) has observed—and as Angus Deaton and Anne Case, Michael Sandel, and other leading scholars have echoed—levels and kinds of inequality that we see in America today reflect a growing divide between the "haves" and "have nots," and levels of dignity that individuals attach to their lives are mirroring these same troubling trends. Dignity is unlikely to be the cause of these divides, but asking about it efficiently *indicates* the lived experience of people in varying positions in society.

Thus, America's political and economic crises are—as we find—reflected in crises of dignity.

## Back to Theory: How Should We Link Dignity Numbers to Dignity Ideas?

Dignity is an evolving product of its own social history. The sheer range of psychological, social, and economic factors correlated with dignity lends support to our contention that dignity draws on many aspects of modern capitalist life. Were Karl Marx, Friedrich Nietzsche, Arthur Schopenhauer, Steven Pinker, and other intellectuals right with their general skepticism toward dignity's social and intellectual value, given the brute conditions we routinely confront in our collective existence as humans, across history's course?

As with love or happiness, we discover dignity in the experience of social relations; we do not ascertain it by logic or reason alone. Hierarchy and power define many of the patterns of dignity we still see today in America. People do not ascertain their own dignities in a vacuum. There is no "us" apart from social processes.

If dignity exists beyond reason, then relationships become much easier to understand as integral forces shaping dignity. By unpacking economic relations inherent to American capitalism, we began to see that historical patterns of wealth and prosperity are underwritten by relations of actual or symbolic violence, and that this violence continues to be experienced through a variety of injustices reflected in dignity levels. While individuals might interpret inequality and discrimination quite differently, this does not wash away the differences in subjective dignity that we see in our analysis. Conversely, not perceiving indignity does not mean it does not exist independently. However, subjective dignity gets at the experience of dignity in ways that objective or structural analysis alone cannot.

Society is never hierarchy-free, but if hierarchy coexists with perceived indignity and associated deficits in health and well-being, then perhaps hierarchy has gone too far. Social capital, or the intricate and wider webs of relationships within which we exist, always carries possible dark sides of promoting or normalizing harmful or deadly behaviors (Coleman 1990; Villalonga-Olives and Kawachi 2017). Such dark webs of connection can be unstable, sowing the seeds of their own destruction. In a world rife with authoritarianism and extreme inequality, improvements do not occur quickly enough. The ongoing existence of inhumane regimes leads to transnational dialogue about dignity and lingering human rights violations. Global institutions and systems shape countries' actions (Habermas 2010; Steinmetz 2014), as nations respond to their reputations in the eyes of other nations, but justice locally and globally remains slow relative to a much longer arc of human suffering.

The particular combination of resources and stress we each live with reflects our positions in society. Advantages are not destiny, nor are disadvantages, but they determine typical outcomes and sources of ease or difficulty. Exceptions do not make the rule, as individuals who defy all odds in order to succeed are not nearly enough to offset the strong patterns we and other researchers have found when it comes to social inequality and its links to health and well-being in America. Because income is disproportionately gained by male, white, able-bodied, and young workers who come from advantaged families, and because income and family background are the primary engines of intergenerational wealth, we do not see our argument as being "political" or "liberal" so much as anchored in average or aggregate economic facts available in confidential tax return data and in labor force data.

Transitioning from these economic and social facts to any moral prescriptions is another issue altogether. Inequalities as phenomena do not provide any straightforward course to telling people what they "should" do (see Hitlin 2021 for an overview). Linking these inequalities to population health, as we have done, provides one compelling warrant for redressing them. If one believes that people all have equal chances and "deserve" what happens to them, thus bracketing structural issues of power or birth location, then one must also say that some individuals deserve to be in poor or ailing health. We do not take that view. Rather, we view dignity as a flashing warning signal that should inform future public health efforts.

## New Knowledge about Dignity: An Efficient Indicator of Fitting into Social and Moral Orders

Our survey items allowed individuals to interpret dignity for themselves. Our measure is similar to self-rated health or to subjective social status in this regard, two leading measures in the epidemiological and medical sciences used by survey researchers who study health and social status (e.g., Andersson 2018a; Idler and Benyamini 1997). These measures allow individuals to interpret social distinctions for themselves by drawing on personalized quantities of information.

By taking this subjective dignity approach, we were able to document several important associations and trends relevant to dignity. What we see is that some of the classically proposed definitional pillars of dignity—such as respect, control, relationships, and financial resources—are empirically associated with subjective levels of dignity. This, in turn, suggests two important things: (1) intellectual or academic understandings of dignity and public, subjective understandings of dignity are overlapping, and (2) what we find about subjective dignity could be relevant to longstanding, theoretical debates about dignity or its nature.

Regarding (1), we cannot claim that individuals were asked explicitly to define dignity. This already has been done in some capacity by some researchers of the concept, such as Lucas (2015), who documented how people talk about workplace dignity. More important, dignity itself is likely subject to moral vocabularies (Lamont and Thévenot 2000) or ways of explaining or justifying action (Swidler 2001): in other words, people have been taught culturally what dignity means in different situations. And when asked to define dignity in general terms, people might be flustered or might contradict themselves, just as Ann Swidler and other researchers of culture and morality have found when people are asked to place their most cherished beliefs about love into words. *In other words, by asking people to define dignity, we are likely to instantiate some of the same conceptual quagmires that brought us here in the first place.*

Even more importantly, many people might have experiences relevant to dignity without labeling them that way. Few people might be likely to think about the word itself—"dignity"—throughout the day, but this does not mean they do not value the concept or experience its meaning. By taking a between-person, correlational approach, we can see what is present in the lives of people who report they have dignity, regardless of whether they would think of certain, specific situations in precisely those terms. By seeing what coincides with dignity from a bird's-eye view, we can learn about what could make for a dignified life across the American lives we surveyed.

How, then, do we make sense of the distinct and changing levels of dignity that we see across different social groups? Because dignity is measured subjectively, at least four processes could be at work: changes in objective circumstances, changing perceptions of those circumstances, changing patterns of coping responses, or changing viewpoints on what dignity means. When we see lower levels of dignity among those who are economically or socially vulnerable, an objective lack of resources likely matters, but we should not discount how individuals change their views of their circumstances in ways that might end up buffering their senses of dignity (Lamont et al. 2016). And while individuals carry a tremendous capability to cope, they still strive for a fair and supportive existence, however they come to define it.

We found that dignity and respect indeed do go together, as do dignity and meaningful social relationships and control over one's life. Crucially, because mastery, meaning, and mattering were not interchangeable with dignity, we can argue that they are not definitionally substitutable concepts. By extension, we could argue that it is unlikely that specific legal conceptions of dignity are interchangeable with dignity universally. Within situations of jurisprudence, case-specific definitions of dignity may be devised in practical terms related to suffering or wrongdoing. This would align with the pragmatic, relational perspective on dignity undergirding our own perspective throughout this book.

Morality itself is a product of concrete situations and the specific codes and emotions they evoke (Hitlin and Vaisey 2013; Luft 2020). Yet, many of the emotions we do experience across many situations relate to our relationships, our felt purpose, and our sense of control. Therefore, our ability to validate these associations with subjective dignity provides evidence that some ingredients of dignity are more important or even are "all-purpose": they seem to cut across many life situations and across many individual lives, like how so many baking recipes call for flour—even as we bake such differing foods. Patterns add up across situations and of course are not incompatible with situational variation.

## Dignity and Health: What Is the Link and What Does It Mean?

By offering an efficient measurement of social and moral integration in American society, subjective dignity could enable new paths forward for population health research. Because it generally is quite expensive to design and implement surveys, the potential for gathering these immense social inputs across just a few simple dignity items is considerable. Given the strengthening associations that we find between depressive symptoms and subjective dignity across the pandemic, it seems plausible that the Covid-19 pandemic is a generalized stressor affecting the population for which dignity might serve as a mental health buffer. Subjective appraisals of life consider time, biography, history, culture, and imagined futures. Dignity survey items hold promise of measurement flexibility across these immense inputs to subjectivity, while also offering a new, robust avenue for relating modern, diverse individualities to health inequities.

For most situations, we favor the interpretation that dignity promotes health. At the same time, we also know that serious health problems can and have undermined people's sense of dignity: through the removal of bodily capacity and thus autonomy, through stigmatization of illness, or through being treated hastily or without dignity during medical treatment, for example. Overall, the nature of the relationship between dignity and health likely depends on the specific health situation (Jacobsen 2007).

Physicians, nurses, aides, families, and stakeholders all attach importance to dignity in health care and dying with dignity (Buchbinder 2021; Jacobsen 2007). Likewise, public health efforts vary in the degree to which they respect or understand the life situations of those whom they target or assist, not just in situations of race and sexual orientation (Engel and Lyle 2021; Watkins-Hayes 2019) but also in situations of Indigenous or native peoples.[1] Recent

---

[1] "Many Native Americans Can't Get Clean Water, Report Finds," NPR Morning Edition, November 18, 2019.

evidence revealing the geographic isolation of American Indian and Alaskan Native populations from radiation therapy underscores not only different ways of treating cancer but also the environmental injustices inherent in exposure to hazardous conditions compounded by a lack of effective treatment for resulting major health problems (Amiri et al. 2022). Analogously, such "spatial mismatches" are routinely documented in major American cities for economic and racial minorities who live far from work or educational opportunities, community resources, or effective, low-cost diabetes treatment (Lutfey and Freese 2005; Wilson 2012).

The pandemic itself is what social scientists would call a natural experiment: it suddenly upended resources, routines, relationships, and even perhaps a sense of control over life. All the while, many people were spared from health problems, even as millions became ill or died within the United States. The fact that subjective dignity decreased significantly and across a variety of groups who remained relatively immune from sudden illness or death likely speaks to dignity's basis in social conditions rather than strictly in health problems. For instance, even well-resourced groups or young groups with relatively lower rates of life-threatening health problems reported sizable losses of dignity. Also, as shown in Chapter 6, individuals with greater levels of dignity in the present expect better health for themselves in the future.

## Resources, Stress, and Polarization: Measuring the Landscape of Dignity in America

There are countless combinations of resources and stress that would lead to the same numeric levels of dignity. This is a provocative and important result speaking to the complexity of lives: pathways, and levels, of dignity are not experienced in the same way, similar to how two individuals who both report being in "good" self-rated health might have differing physical or bodily states.

A key lesson we might take away from this sort of "scientific commensuration" (after Espeland, Sauder, and Espeland 2016; Espeland and Sauder 2007) is that more resources and fewer stressors are generally better for dignity levels, on average, but particularities still do matter, and multiple roads to dignity do and should exist (Lamont 2017). In fact, more institutional, cultural, and economic roads to dignity arguably are needed (Lamont 2019) to repair unraveling subjective dignity levels that we find in this book.

American culture provides, in Lamont's thesis, increasingly few avenues for people to develop enduring senses of dignity.

Because there are multiple paths to dignity, multiple solutions also are likely to exist. However, at the same time, there are non-negotiable basics of dignity: stigma, discrimination, and respect show some of the strongest links to dignity, as do poverty, food insecurity, and membership in several vulnerable groups in society, as we see in this book's findings. Thus, on the whole, it seems fair to say that our dignity findings speak to the simultaneity of structural oppressions and pluralistic forms of social resilience.

If we are convinced that dignity promotion is intricately intertwined with health promotion, then what can we do to change levels of dignity? While it is good news that most Americans "agree" or "strongly agree" that there is dignity in their lives, all levels of dignity associate with health, and many people are neutral or even disagree that there is dignity to their lives. The pandemic only lowered these dignity levels, some to critical lows.

To begin understanding the social roots of dignity, we offered and tested a resource-based explanation. By integrating data on various psychological, economic, and social resources within individual lives, we can make better sense of reported levels of dignity. Indeed, the range of dignity across the range of resources is quite striking. The resource model explains over a quarter of the dignity variation in the population, a strong number in social science, with psychological resources generally demonstrating stronger ties to dignity than economic or social resources. This may not be surprising, as dignity is perceived by individuals, while economic and social resources are more based in external conditions or social environments. And while there is variation in the strength of the resource perspective across different segments of population, it carries significant explanatory value for all groups we studied. Resources matter for dignity no matter which groups we discuss.

Drawing on multidisciplinary inequality perspectives, we positioned a four-year college degree as a generator of many resource differences in society that are psychological, economic, and social. College graduates have higher levels of most of these resources. While the college gap in dignity is not as large as the gap in dignity attached to some of the more potent resources we studied, the fact that a college education so pervasively shapes dignity across numerous resource channel levels speaks to the fundamental (Case and Deaton 2021; Link and Phelan 1995) way that our society has become unequal in wealth, health, and social life according to educational credentials. Because one of the strongest predictors of college attendance and institutional selectivity is whether one's parents went to college, we find that dignity gaps become much larger once combinations of both parental and personal college education are considered.

Helping to chart other ideas for surveying dignity, a recent "beginning college" survey of student engagement found that incoming freshmen are exhausted, speaking to the potential research value of tracking dignity levels during the college experience.[2] Sociological research into school quality similarly finds that where one attends school factors significantly into peer acceptance, support for success, and, most relevantly today, pandemic coping. Students arriving at college these days are living in a state of pandemic exhaustion, and some of this can be traced to (1) the intensive culture of achievement hovering around students that has escalated over the past decades, (2) differences across schools and peer groups, and (3) the particular demands of pandemic learning amid a climate of uncertainty about the future (for frameworks and interventions, see Abelson, Lipson, and Eisenberg 2022; Conley et al. 2017).

An alternative social science model focused on stress-based differences adds to the resource-based explanations for variations in dignity. While stress can erode resources, plenty of individuals experience stress across a variety of resource levels, or even regardless of resources, as the pandemic has made plain. By breaking out numerous Covid-related stressors, such as exposure to the virus, household conflict, food insecurity, delayed health care, pay cuts, and reduced work hours, we learn more about how dignity is distributed in society. Individuals with the least resources endure the most stress, but everyone experiences stress, albeit in different forms. This stems from intersectionality: we all hold multiple statuses across sex, race, class, age, and ability that further shape our stress levels.

A final illustration of dignity variation across political background made the case that dignity matters regardless of one's ideology. Conservatives, moderates, and liberals alike all show strong associations between dignity and respect. Universal associations with health issues show that dignity carries wide importance to understanding well-being within our democracy; to find that resources matter to dignity in a way that ideology cannot erase reminds us of dignity's basis in inequality even if we might disagree about the particulars of the causes or consequences of that inequality. Meanwhile, we also find that polarization bears its own association with dignity levels. In

---

[2] "Incoming Freshmen Are Mentally Exhausted," *Inside Higher Education*, August 17, 2021.

a more polarized society where more of us see more threat from more social groups around us, everyone's dignity suffers.

## Restoring Dignity for Native Peoples

Joy Harjo, American poet laureate, recently stated in an NPR interview, "If my work does nothing else, when I get to the end of my life, I want Native peoples to be seen as human beings." Poetry is the start of an important conversation, as it portrays with striking and relatable immediacy experiences of being left behind, forgotten, or harmed beyond repair. Images and narratives capture dignity where data cannot, and data on dignity reveal trends across lives that can help us in our collective efforts to heal.

Beginning with themes discussed in the emergence of global capitalism in Chapter 4, involving the displacement and social disenfranchisement of native people, and the trends documented in Chapter 9 involving the large decreases in subjective dignity among American Indians from 2017 to 2021, there still is much work to do—and the effects of colonialism linger as a chapter of American history from which native communities might never fully recover.

However, by recognizing that dignity levels are extremely low among Native Americans, and by also recognizing the psychological, economic, and social resources that dictate the distribution of dignity, we might be in a better position to begin to repair our relations. The resource- and stress-based perspectives on dignity make clear that there are many avenues for policymakers to positively impact dignity.

## Religion: A Major Institution for Future Research

Religion is an institutional source of intrinsic dignity, and it also could influence inflorescent dignity through spiritual growth, to go back to Sulmasy's (2007, 2013) dignity framework. The moral communities around which religious practice revolves allow individuals to receive recognition for who they are and the lives they lead, although individuals could experience indignity through a perceived rejection of themselves or their identities within the church. For instance, some denominations have histories of abuse or institutional gender discrimination, while some hold stances on LGBTQ+

individuals that lead to experiences of marginalization. Given our book's emphasis on resource- and stress-based perspectives, there also could be value to exploring how religion shapes levels of psychological, economic, or social resources, or the perception or buffering of stress, in ways that are reflected in ongoing subjective dignity levels. Research by Laura Upenieks (2022) already documents how mental health issues linked to an insecure relationship to God can be offset by perceiving dignity in one's own life. This subjective dignity could have a communal, scriptural, or liturgical basis, or it could come from sources outside the church, representing an important topic for future research into dignity's roots.

## Other Next Steps for Researching Dignity

Dignity has never been more important as a way of imagining social and individual futures. In a structurally unequal world where our categories and bodies prefigure how others might perceive us—where we often rank ourselves and others instead of accepting ourselves and others wholesale—how can we do better? While we tell ourselves stories in order to live and to be understood (McAdams 2013a, 2013b), real knowledge of social inequality could promote cynicism toward feel-good stories.

Growing popular familiarity with "inequality" and "privilege" as cultural terms diffused from the social sciences, and insertion of these same words into personal narratives suggests that a new synthesis between scientific knowledge and individual meaning making could be on the horizon. This could, in turn, represent a shift in how Americans think about dignity, make room for it, and then go about achieving it.

Group-specific or precise underpinnings of dignity remain unclear; a more comprehensive analysis—among the non–college educated, racial or ethnic minorities, women, or the elderly, for instance—could begin to disentangle the effects of having dignity from the broader social conditions supporting dignified lives in the first place. We have discussed this work when it has appeared, largely in qualitative form, but we suggest there is room for much more study. Individuals exist at the intersection of their multiple group identities, making a translation of group-specific findings to individual-level dignity in need of more precise development.

Indeed, an intersectional approach enfolding race, gender, and occupation could provide new insights into how dignity unfolds. Adia Harvey Wingfield

(2019) offers research evidence on Black male nurses who buffer themselves against harassment and microaggressions through their emphasis on the universal importance of care and of the value of each individual they serve. In other words, as Wingfield contends, their moral beliefs supersede categorical distinctions and derive their power from a general valuation of life. This valuation is boundary work, as it occurs in contradistinction to what is perceived as a primary focus on performance or value among whites (see also Lamont 2000).

Applied perspectives on dignity, such as those at the center of political, religious, clinical, or genomic debates, lie mostly beyond the scope of this book. We have referred to them in passing where we can, for illustrative purposes. When people refer to dignity, in such instances, it is often asserted as an a priori good, something obviously positive to strive for. An important lesson for dignity research stems from its anchoring in particular debates. There is no doubt that institutions and the technologies they use will change our experiences of our own individuality and autonomy. A fascinating direction forward for future research would be to begin understanding how subjective dignity varies in response to certain policy stances on gun control, abortion, assisted dying, cloning, or any other controversial issues for which dignity has been mentioned as a grounding concept for positions on different sides of political divides. This could be addressed experimentally using vignette studies or quasi-experimentally through exploiting variation in policy or technological availability.

In our Gallup data, we were unable to track incarcerated individuals. Similarly, the survey did not ask individuals to report any previous incarceration. Building on Devah Pager's groundbreaking audit research into the mark of a criminal record and Bruce Western's work on life after release, incarceration is linked to stigma, health risks, and limited resources both during and after imprisonment. This is an area of dignity research that might be expanded by building on some of the same measurement techniques we use in this book. If we can link up incarceration patterns with inequalities in dignity by race, we might gain more resolution into some of the paradoxical patterns of dignity by race that we uncovered in our data analysis. By learning more about the hardships that are unequal by race, we can decompose dignity into its social determinants.

Another limitation of the approach taken here is that we are focused on adulthood, timed after earlier origins of dignity. Certainly, adverse childhood experiences including abuse or economic hardship growing up have the potential to factor into current dignity levels. Moreover, as the famed life-course sociologist Glen H. Elder Jr. noted when interviewed in a recent piece for *Time* magazine, generational differences reflect past circumstances endured by different generations and how those collective experiences are brought to bear on current patterns of coping and resilience.[3] Current difficulties are linked to perceived trajectories (Frye 2012) and re-evaluated pending later life events. Assessing one's life involves senses of one's past, present, and future (Cerulo and Ruane 2022; Emirbayer and Mische 1998).

Morality, in some fashion, is implicated within the standards people use to ascertain their own sense of dignity, but it is another concept that can be just as complicated as dignity itself. Meanwhile, dignity is clearly patterned by resources and stress. However, if we improve dignity levels by improving levels of resources and mitigating life stress, will we naturally get back to feeling good and doing good for those around us? In fact, there is much to suggest that this assessment is realistic and not optimistic, given how income inequality can undermine moral and social cohesion within societies (Hitlin and Harkness 2018).

Because dignity is determined by numerous factors, where should we start? There is not a clear dignity intervention. However, what we can do is look to where much of the variation in dignity comes from and perhaps start there. Given how staggering resource differences are attached to a college degree, it might be useful to revisit the status attached to college in our society, and to revisit questions of college access and college selectivity. These are economic and social debates well beyond the scope of this book. However, we point out a couple of guideposts here. First, as we mentioned in Chapter 4, there is increasing support for the public or governmental financing of education (Quadlin and Powell 2022). Meanwhile, student debt is a known, prominent obstacle to economic stability during adulthood. Frederick Wherry and colleagues, in their Princeton University Dignity and Debt Network, illustrate how the experience of indebtedness can create obstacles to a dignified life. Financial strain is shaped by income and debt and has been shown by decades of research to erode a sense of control over life and, with this, mental well-being.

Other than working on the fronts of education and debt, we might also continue working on the front of worker pay and respect. Economists have devised careful models of wages and employment, but many predictions

---

[3] Catherine E. Shoichet, "Meet Gen C, the Covid Generation," CNN News, March 11, 2021.

from these models have been overshadowed by the pandemic. When they do try to measure "dignity at work," they suggest that the level of dignity attached to a job matters a great deal to workers; moving from what they term a low-dignity to the highest-dignity job feels equal to workers as much as a 20% increase in wages (Dube, Naidu, and Reich 2022). We still have a lot to learn about how policy and the economy ought to intersect, and few laws are likely to be ironclad. Just like the shape of dignity itself, the shape of the relationship between economy and society is evolving.

The well-worn phrase "earning a living" is quite telling: it speaks to a deep connection between income and life, and alludes to an insidious cultural belief that toil justifies belonging. Why do gender income gaps persist across hundreds of occupations despite the equal levels of education and skill women bring to work? If given the opportunity to have a rewarding career and to raise a family, many people would choose to do both, but some of us are more likely to be forced to choose than others, and women fall into this category far more often than men even within highly educated couples (Cha 2009; England 2010).

Without a doubt, questions of bias and stigma are central to the future of dignity. Saying equal opportunity and providing it are two entirely separate matters, as decades of field experiments have shown (e.g., Correll, In, and Paik 2007; Gaddis 2018; Pager and Shepherd 2008; Pedulla 2018; Quadlin 2018; Quillian et al. 2017). We say what we think people want to hear, but we often do not act accordingly. The third-order nature of bias, as articulated by Cecilia Ridgeway (2019), is that we believe most people think a certain way even if we personally do not. This is enough to create and reinforce the reality that we believe exists. So-called statistical or rational discrimination is caught in this feedback loop between expectations and reality (Tilcsik 2021).

## Subjective Dignity as a Meaningful Sociological Construct

Subjective dignity does not mean that dignity is just an idiosyncratic judgment. If that were the case, we would have expected five empirical results, none of which emerged across all of our analyses: (1) levels of dignity vary evenly, across all levels; (2) social groups do not vary in their dignity; (3) dignity does not predict health; (4) dignity is not patterned by resources or stress; and (5) levels of dignity remain even across the pandemic. By refuting all five of these possibilities, we make a positive case for dignity as a meaningful social construct: dignity is not the absence of meaning; it means something patterned and systematic across thousands of Americans who were randomly selected to participate in Gallup survey research.

At its social worst, expressive individuality paints a narcissistic, bourgeois portrait of perpetual self-therapy and self-discovery in a hostile climate of moral relativism (Bellah et al. 1985). Dignity is consistent with individualism because it rests in autonomy for individuality. Yet, autonomy is a basic, shared need that all of us possess, and social orders with very different criteria for gaining status and worth all have paths to dignity, whether focused more on individualism or collective visions. By being compatible with personal needs and social order, dignity upholds patterns while expressing something fundamental about an individual life well lived.

Declines in some indicators of community involvement have led to the proclamation that we are "still connected" (Fischer 2011; Lee and Bearman 2020) and still show relatively stable levels of trust in others (Schilke, Reimann, and Cook 2021) even if our connections look or feel different than they did before massive urban growth and the digitalization of social life. An increased reliance on personal networks may be one result of this fragmentation, with personal ties serving as a key, "second-personal" basis of affirming who one is and one's worth and humanity more generally.

So, what does Lamont, perhaps the foremost sociological theorist employing the concept, envision as a solution to America's crisis? "One possible way forward," Lamont writes, "is broadening cultural membership by promoting new narratives of hope centered on a plurality of criteria of worth, 'ordinary universalism' and destigmatizing stigmatized groups." Three observations follow: "ordinary universalism" might well be called the universal valuation of individuals, which is the foundation of dignity as a modern, democratic concept. Next, destigmatization represents a key quest of dignity: overcoming obstacles to this universal recognition (negative factors) before promoting growth and extension of potential and skills (positive factors), as the former generally greatly impedes—or sometimes precludes, in cases of severe oppression—the latter. As for the plurality of potential criteria of worth, a recognition of the particularized value systems across groups and their individuals seems quintessential to dignity.[4]

---

[4] The age-old question of whose values are considered normal arises, Lamont suggests, broadening the acceptability but not infinitely; there would still be belief systems considered out of bounds, but those might be limited to ideologies that damage the worth of others.

In *The High Price of Materialism*, Tim Kasser (2003) draws on numerous psychological studies to show how emphasizing consumption and wealth impedes social relationships. This in many ways fortifies the argument of our book: capitalism and its emphasis on consumerism and materialism operate in ways that strain individual dignity. American capitalism in particular shows particularly strong links among work and livelihood. For instance, drawing on thousands of studies motivated by Esping-Andersen's (1990) worlds of welfare capitalism approach, housing, health care, and childcare might be treated by political economies as rights. At the same time, the numerous forms of capitalism present around the world reflect different arrangements involving varying worker protection and rights, flexibility for combining work and family, paid leave, unemployment benefits, and pension plans (Scruggs and Hayes 2017). These affordances, in turn, are related to the stigmatization of unemployment and the stigmatization of taking time off work (Buffel, Beckfield, and Bracke 2017; Williams et al. 2013).

Capitalist ideologies suffuse how we interpret even our most personal experiences. Kristen Neff, a noted psychologist and proponent of self-compassion, might interpret of Lamont's "having" in terms of a fixation on self-esteem or whether one is "good enough," and of Lamont's "being" in terms of what is "good for you" or what allows you to realize or deepen a real relationship with yourself. For instance, how can one validate their experiences and feelings in a way that lends greater legitimacy to their felt needs, rather than treating these needs as being somehow false or unimportant? "Even in the midst of devastation," the meditation teacher Sharon Salzberg wrote (2003, 82), "something within us always points the way to freedom."[5] Rabbi Dr. Samuel Hirsch saw a direct, mutual connection between self-compassion and compassion for others: "That which we love in ourselves, our true human dignity, compels us to recognize and love the same human dignity in all others."[6]

By extension, if society teaches us to see differences rather than similarities, through cultural biases, it stultifies the capacities for self-compassion and compassion toward others. The collective dignity ideology motivating constitutional democracy and transnational human rights projects stands partly opposed to the quantification and evaluation of lives so fundamental to

---

[5] Thank you to T. J. Geiger for posting this quote.

[6] "The Religion of Humanity," an 1853 public lecture delivered by Dr. Samuel Hirsch in Luxembourg. Reprinted in *The Reform Advocate*, a publication edited by Emil G. Hirsch, Chicago, IL, November 13, 1915.

the operation of capitalism and its interlinked structural biases. Defining individuals in terms of differences in performance or value—what they can have or produce, rather than who they are or who they might be—is what Lamont means when she speaks of "moving from having to being" through a creation of heterarchies or alternative systems of human worth that meaningfully countervail economic hierarchies encrusted within our society.

## Some Final Thoughts

In addition to representing a public health concern, the promise of dignity as a concept is impressive: dignity moves us closer to understanding how individuals and societies might relate in ways that preserve and nurture both. Defining dignity is complicated, more practical than abstract, because social life is too.

While this book has not provided definitive answers, it has presented outlines of a scientific framework for thinking about dignity and its undeniable relations to resource-, stress-, and group-related processes. By charting these objective conditions, we can develop objective, scientific understandings of these subjective dignity assessments. Conversely, these subjective assessments might point the way to objective difficulties that can be hard to measure or notice using existing scientific approaches. Some oppressions are felt but not widely recognized.

To conclude, we believe that measuring dignity in America—and hopefully beyond America as well—offers a rare opportunity to understand the complicated, social origins of individual well-being and the real, individual origins of social change.

# References

Abelson, Sara, Sarah Ketchen Lipson, and Daniel Eisenberg. 2022. "Mental Health in College Populations: A Multidisciplinary Review of What Works, Evidence Gaps, and Paths Forward." In *Higher Education: Handbook of Theory and Research*, Vol. 37, edited by Laura W. Perna, 133–238. Springer Nature.

Abend, Gabriel. 2008. "Two Main Problems in the Sociology of Morality." *Theory and Society* 37 (2): 87–125.

Abend, Gabriel. 2013. "What the Science of Morality Doesn't Say about Morality." *Philosophy of the Social Sciences* 43 (2): 157–200.

Abrutyn, Seth, and Omar Lizardo. 2020. "Grief, Care, and Play: Theorizing the Affective Roots of the Social Self." In *Advances in Group Processes*, edited by Shane R. Thye and Edward J. Lawler, 79–108. Emerald Publishing Limited.

Adler, Nancy E., et al. 2000. "Relationship of Subjective and Objective Social Status with Psychological and Objective Functioning: Preliminary Data in Healthy, White Women." *Health Psychology* 19 (6): 586–92.

Adler, Nancy E., and Jacinth J. X. Tan. 2017. "Tackling the Health Gap: The Role of Psychosocial Processes." *International Journal of Epidemiology* 46 (4): 1329–31.

Albers, Josef. 2013. *Interaction of Color*. Yale University Press.

Alexander, Michelle. 2011. "The New Jim Crow." *Ohio State Journal of Criminal Law* 9: 7.

Alon, Sigal, and Marta Tienda. 2007. "Diversity, Opportunity, and the Shifting Meritocracy in Higher Education." *American Sociological Review* 72 (4): 487–511.

Alwin, Duane F., Ronald L. Cohen, and Theodore M. Newcomb. 1991. *Political Attitudes over the Life Span: The Bennington Women after Fifty Years*. Madison: University of Wisconsin Press.

Amiri, Solmaz, Matthew D. Greer, Clemma J. Muller, Patrik Johansson, Anthippy Petras, Cole C. Allick, Sara M. London, Morgan C. Abbey, Lia M. Halasz, and Dedra S. Buchwald. 2022. "Disparities in Access to Radiation Therapy by Race and Ethnicity in the United States with Focus on American Indian/Alaska Native People." *Value in Health* 25 (12): 1929–38.

Andersen, Susan M., and Serena Chen. 2002. "The Relational Self: An Interpersonal Social-Cognitive Theory." *Psychological Review* 109 (4): 619–45.

Anderson, Elijah. 2022. *Black in White Space: The Enduring Impact of Color in Everyday Life*. University of Chicago Press.

Anderson, Kathryn Freeman, and Darra Ray-Warren. 2022. "Racial-Ethnic Residential Clustering and Early COVID-19 Vaccine Allocations in Five Urban Texas Counties." *Journal of Health and Social Behavior* 63 (4): 472–90.

Anderson, Leon, and David A. Snow. 2001. "Inequality and the Self: Exploring Connections from an Interactionist Perspective." *Symbolic Interaction* 24: 395–406.

Andersson, Matthew A. 2012. "Dispositional Optimism and the Emergence of Social Network Diversity." *Sociological Quarterly* 53 (1): 92–115.

Andersson, Matthew A. 2018a. "An Odd Ladder to Climb: Socioeconomic Differences across Levels of Subjective Social Status." *Social Indicators Research* 136 (2): 621–43.

Andersson, Matthew A. 2018b. "Against All Odds or by Dint of Privilege? Happiness and Life Satisfaction Returns to College in America." *Socius* 4: 2378023118773158.

Andersson, Matthew A. 2022. "Seeing Class in Ladders: An Integrated Approach to Subjective Status and Health Inequality." *Sociological Perspectives* 65 (3): 608–29.

Andersson, Matthew A., Michael A. Garcia, and Jennifer Glass. 2021. "Work–Family Reconciliation and Children's Well-Being Disparities across OECD Countries." *Social Forces* 100 (2): 794–820.

Andersson, Matthew A., and Catherine E. Harnois. 2020. "Higher Exposure, Lower Vulnerability? The Curious Case of Education, Gender Discrimination, and Women's Health." *Social Science & Medicine* 246: 112780.

Andersson, Matthew A., and Steven Hitlin. 2022. "Subjective Dignity and Self-Reported Health: Results from the United States before and during the Covid-19 Pandemic." *SSM-Mental Health* 2: 100113.

Ansari, Arya, and Robert C. Pianta. 2018. "Variation in the Long-Term Benefits of Child Care: The Role of Classroom Quality in Elementary School." *Developmental Psychology* 54 (10): 1854.

Archer, Margaret. 2007. *Making Our Way through the World: Human Reflexivity and Social Mobility*. New York: Cambridge University Press.

Atuahene, Bernadette. 2016. "Dignity Takings and Dignity Restoration: Creating a New Theoretical Framework for Understanding Involuntary Property Loss and the Remedies Required." *Law & Social Inquiry* 41 (4): 796–823.

Bagaric, Mirko, and James Allan. 2006. "The Vacuous Concept of Dignity." *Journal of Human Rights* 5 (2): 257–70. doi:10.1080/14754830600653603.

Bandura, Albert. 1977. "Self-Efficacy: Toward a Unifying Theory of Behavioral Change." *Psychological Review* 84 (2): 191.

Bargheer, Stefan. 2018. *Moral Entanglements: Conserving Birds in Britain and Germany*. University of Chicago Press.

Bellah, Robert, Richard Madsen, William M. Sullivan, Ann Swidler, and Steven M. Tipton, eds. 1985. *Habits of the Heart Individualism and Commitment in American Life*. Berkeley: University of California Press.

Berger, Peter. 1970. "On the Obsolescence of the Concept of Honor." *European Journal of Sociology/Archives Européennes de Sociologie* 11 (2): 338–47.

Berger, Peter L., and Thomas Luckmann. 1966. *The Social Construction of Reality*. Garden City, NY: Anchor.

Berghammer, Caroline, and Melissa A. Milkie. 2021. "Felt Deficits in Time with Children: Individual and Contextual Factors across 27 European Countries." *British Journal of Sociology* 72 (5): 1168–99.

Berman, Elizabeth Popp. 2022. *Thinking Like an Economist: How Efficiency Replaced Equality in US Public Policy*. Princeton University Press.

Berreby, David. 2005. *Us and Them: Understanding Your Tribal Mind*. New York: Little, Brown, and Co.

Binder, Amy J., Daniel B. Davis, and Nick Bloom. 2016. "Career Funneling: How Elite Students Learn to Define and Desire 'Prestigious' Jobs." *Sociology of Education* 89 (1): 20–39.

Biss, Eula. 2020. *Having and Being Had*. New York: Riverhead Books.

Black, Donald. 2002. "Pure Sociology and the Geometry of Discovery." *Contemporary Sociology* 31: 668–74.

Blair-Loy, Mary. 2003. *Competing Devotions: Career and Family among Women Executives.* Cambridge, MA: Harvard University Press.

Bloome, Deirdre. 2017. "Childhood Family Structure and Intergenerational Income Mobility in the United States." *Demography* 54 (2): 541–69.

Bloome, Deirdre, Shauna Dyer, and Xiang Zhou. 2018. "Educational Inequality, Educational Expansion, and Intergenerational Income Persistence in the United States." *American Sociological Review* 83 (6): 1215–53.

Blumer, Herbert. 1969. *Symbolic Interactionism: Perspective Method.* Englewood Cliffs, NJ: Prentice Hall.

Bolton, Sharon, ed. 2007. *Dimensions of Dignity at Work.* London: Routledge.

Bonilla-Silva, Eduardo. 2010. *Racism without Racists.* New York: Rowman & Littlefield.

Bourdieu, Pierre. 1984. *Distinction: A Social Critique of the Judgement of Taste.* Cambridge, MA: Harvard University Press.

Bourdieu, Pierre. 1986. "The Forms of Capital." In *Handbook of Theory and Research for the Sociology of Education,* edited by J. G. Richardson, 241–58. New York: Greenwood.

Bourdieu, Pierre. 1990. *The Logic of Practice.* Stanford University Press.

Bourgois, Philippe. 2003. *In Search of Respect: Selling Crack in El Barrio.* Cambridge: Cambridge University Press.

Boutyline, Andrei, and Stephen Vaisey. 2017. "Belief Network Analysis: A Relational Approach to Understanding the Structure of Attitudes." *American Journal of Sociology* 122 (5): 1371–447.

Brennan, Andrew, and Y. S. Lo. 2007. "Two Conceptions of Dignity: Honour and Self-Determination." In *Perspectives on Human Dignity: A Conversation,* edited by Jeff Malpas and Norelle Lickiss, 43–58. New York: Springer.

Brubaker, Rogers, and Frederick Cooper. 2000. "Beyond Identity." *Theory and Society* 29 (1): 1–47.

Buchanan, Allen, and Russell Powell. 2018. *The Evolution of Moral Progress: A Biocultural Theory.* Oxford University Press.

Buchbinder, Mara. 2021. *Scripting Death.* Oakland: University of California Press.

Buffel, Veerle, Jason Beckfield, and Piet Bracke. 2017. "The Institutional Foundations of Medicalization: A Cross-National Analysis of Mental Health and Unemployment." *Journal of Health and Social Behavior* 58 (3): 272–90.

Burke, Peter J., and Jan E. Stets. 2009. *Identity Theory.* Oxford University Press.

Byk, Judge Christian. 2014. "Is Human Dignity a Useless Concept? Legal Perspectives." In *Cambridge Handbook on Human Dignity,* edited by M. Düwell, J. Braarvig, R. Brownsword, and D. Mieth, 362–67. Cambridge: Cambridge University Press.

Cabanas, Edgar, and Eva Illouz. 2019. *Manufacturing Happy Citizens: How the Science and Industry of Happiness Control Our Lives.* John Wiley & Sons.

Cahill, Spencer E. 1998. "Toward a Sociology of the Person." *Sociological Theory* 16 (2): 131–48.

Calarco, Jessica McCrory. 2014. "Coached for the Classroom Parents' Cultural Transmission and Children's Reproduction of Educational Inequalities." *American Sociological Review* 79 (5): 1015–37.

Calarco, Jessica McCrory. 2018. *Negotiating Opportunities: How the Middle Class Secures Advantages in School.* Oxford University Press.

Calhoun, Craig. 1991. "Morality, Identity, and Historical Explanation: Charles Taylor on the Sources of the Self." *Sociological Theory* 9 (2): 232–63.

Callero, Peter L. 2003. "The Sociology of the Self." *Annual Review of Sociology* 29: 115–33.

Callero, Peter L. 2014. "Self, Identity, and Social Inequality." In *Handbook of the Social Psychology of Inequality*, edited by Jane McLeod, Michael Schwalbe, and Ed Lawler, 273–94. New York: Springer.

Callero, Peter L. 2018. *Being Unequal: How Identity Helps Make and Break Power and Privilege*. Boulder, CO: Rowman & Littlefield.

Camic, Charles. 1986. "The Matter of Habit." *American Journal of Sociology* 91 (5): 1039–87.

Campos-Castillo, Celeste, and Steven Hitlin. 2013. "Copresence Revisiting a Building Block for Social Interaction Theories." *Sociological Theory* 31 (2): 168–92.

Cannon, Bryan C., Dawn T. Robinson, and Lynn Smith-Lovin. 2019. "How Do We 'Do Gender'? Permeation as Over-Talking and Talking Over." *Socius* 5: 2378023119849347.

Carlson, Daniel L., Richard J. Petts, and Joanna R. Pepin. 2021. "Changes in US Parents' Domestic Labor during the Early Days of the COVID-19 Pandemic." *Sociological Inquiry* 92 (3): 1217–44.

Carr, Deborah, and Eun Ha Namkung. 2021. "Physical Disability at Work: How Functional Limitation Affects Perceived Discrimination and Interpersonal Relationships in the Workplace." *Journal of Health and Social Behavior* 62 (4): 545–61.

Case, A., and A. Deaton. 2021. *Deaths of Despair and the Future of Capitalism*. Princeton, NJ: Princeton University Press.

Cech, Erin. 2021. *The Trouble with Passion: How Searching for Fulfillment at Work Fosters Inequality*. Oakland: University of California Press.

Cech, Erin A., and Mary Blair-Loy. 2010. "Perceiving Glass Ceilings? Meritocratic versus Structural Explanations of Gender Inequality among Women in Science and Technology." *Social Problems* 57 (3): 371–97.

Cerulo, Karen A. 2010. "Mining the Intersections of Cognitive Sociology and Neuroscience." *Poetics* 38: 115–32.

Cerulo, Karen A., and Janet M. Ruane. 2022. *Dreams of a Lifetime: How Who We Are Shapes How We Imagine Our Future*. Princeton, NJ: Princeton University Press.

Cha, Youngjoo. 2009. "Reinforcing Separate Spheres: The Effect of Spousal Overwork on the Employment of Men and Women in Dual-Earner Households." *American Sociological Review* 75 (2): 303–29.

Chang, Virginia W., and Diane S. Lauderdale. 2009. "Fundamental Cause Theory, Technological Innovation, and Health Disparities: The Case of Cholesterol in the Era of Statins." *Journal of Health and Social Behavior* 50 (3): 245–60.

Chetty, Raj, et al. 2017. "The Fading American Dream: Trends in Absolute Income Mobility since 1940." *Science* 356 (6336): 398–406.

Christakis, Nicholas A. 2007. "The Social Origins of Dignity in Medical Care at the End of Life." In *Perspectives on Human Dignity: A Conversation*, edited by Jeff Malpas and Norelle Lickiss, 199–208. New York: Springer.

Chun, Hyunsik, and Michael Sauder. 2022. "The Logic of Quantification: Institutionalizing Numerical Thinking." *Theory and Society* 51: 335–70.

Clair, Matthew, Caitlin Daniel, and Michèle Lamont. 2016. "Destigmatization and Health: Cultural Constructions and the Long-Term Reduction of Stigma." *Social Science & Medicine* 165: 223–32.

Coleman, James S. 1988. "Social Capital in the Creation of Human Capital." *American Journal of Sociology* 94: S95–120.

Commonwealth Fund. 2021. "Meeting the Health Care Needs of Transgender People without Housing." Research Report, November 5.

Conley, Colleen S., et al. 2017. "A Meta-Analysis of Indicated Mental Health Prevention Programs for At-Risk Higher Education Students." *Journal of Counseling Psychology* 64 (2): 121.

Cooley, Charles Horton, ed. 1902. *Human Nature and the Social Order.* New York: Scribner.

Correll, Shelley J. 2001. "Gender and the Career Choice Process: The Role of Biased Self-Assessments." *American Journal of Sociology* 106 (6): 1691–730.

Correll, Shelley J. 2004. "Constraints into Preferences: Gender, Status, and Emerging Career Aspirations." *American Sociological Review* 69 (1): 93–113.

Correll, Shelley J., Stephen Benard, and In Paik. 2007. "Getting a Job: Is There a Motherhood Penalty?" *American Journal of Sociology* 112 (5): 1297–338.

Crimston, Charlie R., Matthew J. Hornsey, Paul G. Bain, and Brock Bastian. 2018. "Toward a Psychology of Moral Expansiveness." *Current Directions in Psychological Science* 27 (1): 14–19.

Crowley, Martha. 2013. "Gender, the Labor Process and Dignity at Work." *Social Forces* 91: 1209–38.

Crowley, Martha. 2014. "Class, Control, and Relational Indignity: Labor Process Foundations for Workplace Humiliation, Conflict, and Shame." *American Behavioral Scientist* 58: 416–34.

Cuddy, Amy J. C., Susan T. Fiske, and Peter Glick. 2004. "When Professionals Become Mothers, Warmth Doesn't Cut the Ice." *Journal of Social Issues* 60 (4): 701–18.

Cundiff, Jenny M., and Karen A. Matthews. 2017. "Is Subjective Social Status a Unique Correlate of Physical Health? A Meta-Analysis." *Health Psychology* 36 (12): 1109.

Damasio, Antonio R. 1994. "Descartes' Error and the Future of Human Life." *Scientific American* 271 (4): 144.

Damasio, Antonio. 1999. *The Feeling of What Happens.* San Diego: Harcourt.

Dan-Cohen, Meir. 2011. "A Concept of Dignity." *Israel Law Review* 44 (1–2): 9–23. doi:10.1017/s0021223700000947.

Darwall, Stephen. 2017. "Equal Dignity and Rights." In *Dignity*, edited by R. Debes, 181–202. New York: Oxford University Press.

Debes, Remy. 2009. "Dignity's Gauntlet." *Philosophical Perspectives* 23 (1): 45–78.

Debes, Remy. 2017a. "Human Dignity before Kant: Denis Diderot's Passionate Person." In *Dignity*, edited by R. Debes, 203–36. New York: Oxford University Press.

Debes, Remy. 2017b. *Dignity: A History.* Oxford University Press.

Deci, Edward L., and Richard M. Ryan. 2000. "The 'What' and 'Why' of Goal Pursuits: Human Needs and the Self-Determination of Behavior." *Psychological Inquiry* 11 (4): 227–68.

Desmond, Matthew. 2012. "Eviction and the Reproduction of Urban Poverty." *American Journal of Sociology* 118 (1): 88–133.

DiPrete, Thomas A., and Claudia Buchmann. 2013. *The Rise of Women: The Growing Gender Gap in Education and What It Means for American Schools.* Russell Sage Foundation.

DiPrete, Thomas A., and Gregory M. Eirich. 2006. "Cumulative Advantage as a Mechanism for Inequality: A Review of Theoretical and Empirical Developments." *Annual Review of Sociology* 32: 271–97.

Douzinas, Costas. 2002. "Identity, Recognition, Rights or What Can Hegel Teach Us about Human Rights?" *Journal of Law and Society* 29 (3): 379–405.

Dube, Arindrajit, Suresh Naidu, and Adam D. Reich. 2022. *Power and Dignity in the Low-Wage Labor Market: Theory and Evidence from Wal-Mart Workers*. No. w30441. National Bureau of Economic Research.

Duckworth, Angela L., et al. 2007. "Grit: Perseverance and Passion for Long-Term Goals." *Journal of Personality and Social Psychology* 92 (6): 1087.

Durkheim, Emile. 1972. *Emile Durkheim: Selected Writings*. Edited and translated by Anthony Giddens. New York: Cambridge University Press.

Düwell, Marcus. 2014. "Human Dignity: Concept, Discussions, Philosophical Perspectives: Interdisciplinary Perspectives." In *Cambridge Handbook on Human Dignity*, edited by M. Düwell, J. Braarvig, R. Brownsword, and D. Mieth, 23–49. Cambridge: Cambridge University Press.

Düwell, Marcus, Jens Braarvig, Roger Brownsword, and Dietmar Mieth. 2014. *The Cambridge Handbook of Human Dignity: Interdisciplinary Perspectives*. Cambridge University Press.

Dworkin, Ronald. 2006. *Is Democracy Possible Here?* Princeton, NJ: Princeton University Press.

Elder Jr., Glen H. 1994. "Time, Human Agency, and Social Change: Perspectives on the Life Course." *Social Psychology Quarterly* 57 (1): 4–15.

Eliasoph, Nina, and Paul Lichterman. 2003. "Culture in Interaction." *American Journal of Sociology* 108 (4): 735–94.

Emirbayer, Mustafa. 1997. "Manifesto for a Relational Sociology." *American Journal of Sociology* 103 (2): 281–317.

Emirbayer, Mustafa, and Jeff Goodwin. 1994. "Network Analysis, Culture, and the Problem of Agency." *American Journal of Sociology* 99 (6): 1411–54.

Emirbayer, Mustafa, and Ann Mische. 1998. "What Is Agency?" *American Journal of Sociology* 103 (4): 962–1023.

Engel, Stephen M., and Timothy S. Lyle. 2021. *Disrupting Dignity: Rethinking Power and Progress within LGBTQ Lives*. New York: New York University Press.

England, Paula. 2010. "The Gender Revolution: Uneven and Stalled." *Gender & Society* 24 (2): 149–66.

Espeland, Wendy Nelson, and Michael Sauder. 2007. "Rankings and Reactivity: How Public Measures Recreate Social Worlds." *American Journal of Sociology* 113: 1–40.

Espeland, Wendy Nelson, Michael Sauder, and Wendy Espeland. 2016. *Engines of Anxiety: Academic Rankings, Reputation, and Accountability*. New York: Russell Sage Foundation.

Esping-Andersen, Gosta. 1990. *The Three Worlds of Welfare Capitalism*. Princeton University Press.

Fan, Wen, Yue Qian, and Yongai Jin. 2021. "Stigma, Perceived Discrimination, and Mental Health during China's COVID-19 Outbreak: A Mixed-Methods Investigation." *Journal of Health and Social Behavior* 62 (4): 562–81.

Farkas, George. 2018. "Family, Schooling, and Cultural Capital." In *Handbook of the Sociology of Education in the 21st Century*, edited by Barbara Schneider, 3–38. New York: Springer.

Farmer, Paul, et al. 2013. *Reimagining Global Health: An Introduction*. Vol. 26. University of California Press.

Ferraro, Kenneth F. 2018. *The Gerontological Imagination: An Integrative Paradigm of Aging*. Oxford University Press.

Ferraro, Kenneth F., Tetyana Pylypiv Shippee, and Markus H. Schafer. 2009. "Cumulative Inequality Theory for Research on Aging and the Life Course."

Ferraro, Kenneth F., Markus H. Schafer, and Lindsay R. Wilkinson. 2016. "Childhood Disadvantage and Health Problems in Middle and Later Life: Early Imprints on Physical Health?" *American Sociological Review* 81 (1): 107–33.

Firat, Rengin, and Steven Hitlin. 2012. "Morally Bonded and Bounded: A Sociological Introduction to Neurology." *Biosociology and Neurosociology* 29: 165–99.

Fischer, Claude S. 2011. *Still Connected: Family and Friends in America Since 1970*. New York: Russell Sage Foundation.

Fiske, Susan. 2004. "Intent and Ordinary Bias: Unintended Thought and Social Motivation Create Casual Prejudice." *Social Justice Research* 17: 117–27.

Franks, David D. 2010. *Neurosociology: The Nexus between Neuroscience and Social Psychology*. Springer Science & Business Media.

Freese, Jeremy, and Karen Lutfey. 2011. "Fundamental Causality: Challenges of an Animating Concept for Medical Sociology." In *Handbook of the Sociology of Health, Illness, and Healing*, edited by Bernice A. Pescosolido, Jack K. Martin, Jane D. McLeod, and Anne Rogers, 67–81. New York: Springer.

Frye, Margaret T. 2012. "Bright Futures in Malawi's New Dawn: Educational Aspirations as Assertions of Identity." *American Journal of Sociology* 117 (6): 1565–624.

Frye, Margaret T. 2019. "The Myth of Agency and the Misattribution of Blame in Collective Imaginaries of the Future." *British Journal of Sociology* 70: 721–30.

Gaddis, S. Michael. 2018. "An Introduction to Audit Studies in the Social Sciences." In *Audit Studies: Behind the Scenes with Theory, Method, and Nuance*, edited by S. Michael Gaddis, 3–44. New York: Springer.

Garcia, Marc A., et al. 2021. "The Color of COVID-19: Structural Racism and the Disproportionate Impact of the Pandemic on Older Black and Latinx Adults." *Journals of Gerontology: Series B* 76 (3): e75–80.

Garfinkel, Harold. 1967. *Studies in Ethnomethodology*. Englewood Cliffs, NJ: Prentice-Hall.

Gates, Melinda. 2019. *The Moment of Lift: How Empowering Women Changes the World*. Flatiron Books.

Gauchat, Gordon. 2015. "The Political Context of Science in the United States: Public Acceptance of Evidence-Based Policy and Science Funding." *Social Forces* 94 (2): 723–46.

Gay, Roxane. 2014. *Bad Feminist: Essays*. New York: HarperCollins.

Gecas, Viktor. 2003. "Self-Agency and the Life Course." In *Handbook of the Life Course*, edited by J. T. Mortimer and M. Shanahan, 369–88. New York: Klewer.

Gelfand, Michèle J., et al. 2011. "Differences between Tight and Loose Cultures: A 33-Nation Study." *Science* 332 (6033): 1100–104.

Geronimus, Arline T., et al. 2019. "Weathering, Drugs, and Whack-a-Mole: Fundamental and Proximate Causes of Widening Educational Inequity in US Life Expectancy by Sex and Race, 1990–2015." *Journal of Health and Social Behavior* 60 (2): 222–39.

Gerth, Hans Heinrich, and Charles Wright Mills. 1953. *Character and Social Structure: The Psychology of Social Institutions*. New York: Harcourt, Brace.

Giddens, Anthony, ed. 1984. *The Constitution of Society Introduction of the Theory of Structuration*. Berkeley: University of California Press.

Giddens, Anthony. 1991. *Modernity and Self-Identity: Self and Society in the Late Modern Age*. New York: Polity.

Gigerenzer, Gerd. 2010. "Moral Satisficing: Rethinking Moral Behavior as Bounded Rationality." *Topics in Cognitive Science* 2 (3): 528–54.

Glass, Jennifer, Robin W. Simon, and Matthew A. Andersson. 2016. "Parenthood and Happiness: Effects of Work-Family Reconciliation Policies in 22 OECD Countries." *American Journal of Sociology* 122 (3): 886–929.

Goffman, Erving, ed. 1959. *The Presentation of Self in Everyday Life*. Garden City, NY: Doubleday.

Goffman, Erving. 1963. *Stigma: Notes on the Management of Spoiled Identity*. New York: Simon & Shuster.

Goffman, Erving. 1967. *Interaction Ritual*. New York: Anchor Books.

Goffman, Erving, ed. 1974. *Frame Analysis: An Essay on the Organization of Experience*. New York: Harper & Row.

Goffman, Erving. 1983. "The Interaction Order: American Sociological Association, 1982 Presidential Address." *American Sociological Review* 48 (1): 1–17.

Goldin, Claudia. 2014. "A Grand Gender Convergence: Its Last Chapter." *American Economic Review* 104: 1091–119.

Granovetter, Mark. 1985. "Economic Action and Social Structure: The Problem of Embeddedness." *American Journal of Sociology* 91: 481–510.

Gray, Kurt, and Jesse Graham, eds. 2018. *The Model of Moral Motives*. New York: Guilford.

Greene, Joshua. 2013. *Moral Tribes: Emotion, Reason, and the Gap between Us and Them*. New York: Penguin.

Grollman, Eric Anthony. 2012. "Multiple Forms of Perceived Discrimination and Health among Adolescents and Young Adults." *Journal of Health and Social Behavior* 53 (2): 199–214.

Grusky, David, and Jasmine Hill, eds. 2018. *Inequality in the 21st Century: A Reader*. Routledge.

Guhin, Jeffrey, Jessica McCrory Calarco, and Cynthia Miller-Idriss. 2021. "Whatever Happened to Socialization?" *Annual Review of Sociology* 47: 109–29.

Habermas, Jurgen. 2010. "The Concept of Human Dignity and the Realistic Utopia of Human Rights." *Metaphilosophy* 41 (4): 464–80.

Haidt, Jonathan. 2001. "The Emotional Dog and Its Rational Tail: A Social Intuitionist Approach to Moral Judgement." *Psychological Review* 108 (4): 814–34.

Haidt, Jonathan. 2006. *The Happiness Hypothesis*. New York: Basic Books.

Haidt, Jonathan, and Judith Rodin. 1999. "Control and Efficacy as Interdisciplinary Bridges." *Review of General Psychology* 3 (4): 317–37.

Hall, P. A., and M. Lamont, eds. 2013. *Social Resilience in the Neoliberal Era*. Cambridge University Press.

Hanushek, Eric A. 2009. "Building on No Child Left Behind." *Science* 326 (5954): 802–3.

Healy, Kieran. 2017. "Fuck Nuance." *Sociological Theory* 35 (2): 118–27.

Hearn, James C. 1991. "Academic and Nonacademic Influences on the College Destinations of 1980 High School Graduates." *Sociology of Education* 64 (3): 158–71.

Hecht, Jennifer Michael. 2013. *Stay: A History of Suicide and the Philosophies against It*. Yale University Press.

Heckman, James J. 2006. "Skill Formation and the Economics of Investing in Disadvantaged Children." *Science* 312 (5782): 1900–1902.

Heckman, James J., and Alan B. Krueger. 2003. *Inequality in America: What Role for Human Capital Policies?* Cambridge, MA: MIT Press.

Hegtvedt, Karen A. 2006. "Justice Frameworks." In *Contemporary Social Psychological Theories*, edited by P. J. Burke, 46–69. Stanford, CA: Stanford University Press.

Heinz, Walter R. 2002. "Self-Socialization and Post-Traditional Society." In *Advances in Life Course Research*, Vol. 7, edited by R. A. Settersten Jr. and T. J. Owens, 41–64. JAI Press.

Hewitt, John P. 1997. *Self and Society: A Symbolic Interactionist Social Psychology*. Boston: Allyn and Bacon.

Hicks, Donna. 2011. *Dignity: Its Essential Role in Resolving Conflict*. New York: Yale University Press.

Hitlin, Steven. 2003. "Values as the Core of Personal Identity: Drawing Links between Two Theories of the Self." *Social Psychology Quarterly* 66 (2): 118–37.

Hitlin, Steven. 2008. *Moral Selves, Evil Selves: The Social Psychology of Conscience*. New York: Palgrave Macmillan.

Hitlin, Steven. 2021. "Morality and Sociological Theory." In *Handbook of Classical Sociological Theory*, edited by Seth Abrutyn and Omar Lizardo, 631–49. New York: Springer.

Hitlin, Steven, and Matthew A. Andersson. 2013. "Dignity." In *Handbook of Sociology and Human Rights*, edited by D. L. Brunsma, K. E. I. Smith, and B. K. Bran, 384–93. Boulder, CO: Paradigm.

Hitlin, Steven, and Matthew A. Andersson. 2015. "Dignity as Moral Motivation: The Problem of Social Order Writ Small." In *Order on the Edge of Chaos: Social Psychology and the Problem of Social Order*, edited by E. J. Lawler, S. R. Thye, and J. Yoon, 268–85. New York: Cambridge University Press.

Hitlin, Steven, and Glen H. Elder Jr. 2007. "Understanding 'Agency': Clarifying a Curiously Abstract Concept." *Sociological Theory* 25 (2): 170–91.

Hitlin, Steven, and Sarah K. Harkness. 2018. *Unequal Foundations: Inequality, Morality, and Emotions across Cultures*. Oxford University Press.

Hitlin, Steven, and Monica Kirkpatrick Johnson. 2015. "Reconceptualizing Agency within the Life Course: The Power of Looking Ahead." *American Journal of Sociology* 120 (5): 1429–72.

Hitlin, Steven, and Charisse Long. 2009. "Agency as a Sociological Variable: A Preliminary Model of Individuals, Situations, and the Life Course." Sociology Compass 3 (1): 137–60.

Hitlin, Steven, and Jane Allyn Piliavin. 2004. "Values: Reviving a Dormant Concept." *Annual Review of Sociology* 30: 359–93.

Hitlin, Steven, and Mark H. Salisbury. 2013. "Living Life for Others and/or Oneself: The Social Development of Life Orientations." *Social Science Research* 42 (6): 1622–34.

Hitlin, Steven, and Stephen Vaisey. 2013. "The New Sociology of Morality." *Annual Review of Sociology* 39: 51–68.

Hochschild, Arlie Russell. 1979. "Emotion Work, Feeling Rules, and Social Structure." *American Journal of Sociology* 85 (3): 551–75.

Hodgkiss, Philip. 2013. "A Moral Vision: Human Dignity in the Eyes of the Founders of Sociology." *Sociological Review* 61 (3): 417–39. doi:10.1111/1467-954x.12049.

Hodgkiss, Philip. 2015. "The Origins of the Idea and Ideal of Dignity in the Sociology of Work and Employment." In *The Sage Handbook of the Sociology of Work and Employment*, edited by Edward Granter, Heidi Gottfried, and Stephen Edgell, 129–47. New York: Sage.

Hodgkiss, Philip. 2018. *Social Thought and Rival Claims to the Moral Ideal of Dignity*. New York: Anthem Press.

Hodson, Randy. 1996. "Dignity in the Workplace under Participative Management: Alienation and Freedom Revisited." *American Sociological Review* 61: 719–38.

Hodson, Randy. 2001. *Dignity at Work*. Cambridge: Cambridge University Press.

Hodson, Randy, and Vincent J. Roscigno. 2004. "Organizational Success and Worker Dignity: Complementary or Contradictory?" *American Journal of Sociology* 110: 672–708.

Hojman, Daniel A., and Álvaro Miranda. 2018. "Agency, Human Dignity, and Subjective Well-Being." *World Development* 101: 1–15.

Homan, Patricia. 2019. "Structural Sexism and Health in the United States: A New Perspective on Health Inequality and the Gender System." *American Sociological Review* 84 (3): 486–516.

Houle, Jason N. 2014. "A Generation Indebted: Young Adult Debt across Three Cohorts." *Social Problems* 61 (3): 448–65.

Hout, Michael. 2012. "Social and Economic Returns to College Education in the United States." *Annual Review of Sociology* 38 (1): 379–400.

Hsieh, Ning, and stef m. shuster. 2021. "Health and Health Care of Sexual and Gender Minorities." *Journal of Health and Social Behavior* 62 (3): 318–33.

Hunt, Matthew O., Pamela Braboy Jackson, Samuel H. Kye, Brian Powell, and Lala Carr Steelman. 2013. "Still Color-Blind? The Treatment of Race, Ethnicity, Intersectionality, and Sexuality in Sociological Social Psychology." In *Advances in Group Processes*, 21–45. Bingley, UK: Emerald Group Publishing Limited.

Hunt, Matthew O., Paul R. Croll, and Maria Krysan. 2022. "Public Beliefs about the Black/White Socioeconomic Status Gap: What's 'Upbringing' Got to Do with It?" *Social Science Quarterly* 103 (1): 82–89.

Hunter, James Davison. 2000. *The Death of Character: Moral Education after the Death of God*. New York: Basic Books.

Idler, Ellen L., and Yael Benyamini. 1997. "Self-Rated Health and Mortality: A Review of Twenty-Seven Community Studies." *Journal of Health and Social Behavior* 38 (1): 21–37.

Idler, Ellen, and Kate Cartwright. 2018. "What Do We Rate When We Rate Our Health? Decomposing Age-Related Contributions to Self-Rated Health." *Journal of Health and Social Behavior* 59 (1): 74–93.

Inglehart, Ronald, and Christian Welzel. 2005. *Modernization, Cultural Change, and Democracy*. New York: Cambridge University Press.

Inkeles, Alex. 1969. "Making Men Modern: On the Causes and Consequences of Individual Change in Six Developing Countries." *American Journal of Sociology* 75 (2): 208–25.

Jackson, Margot I. 2015. "Cumulative Inequality in Child Health and Academic Achievement." *Journal of Health and Social Behavior* 56 (2): 262–80.

James, William, ed. 1892. *The Self*. Cleveland, OH: World Publishing.

Janke, Alexander T., et al. 2021. "Analysis of Hospital Resource Availability and COVID-19 Mortality across the United States." *Journal of Hospital Medicine* 16 (4): 211–14.

Jerrim, John, and Lindsey Macmillan. 2015. "Income Inequality, Intergenerational Mobility, and the Great Gatsby Curve: Is Education the Key?" *Social Forces* 94 (2): 505–33.

Joas, Hans. 1996. *The Creativity of Action*. Chicago: University of Chicago Press.

Joas, Hans, ed. 2000. *The Genesis of Values*. Cambridge: Polity Press.

Joas, Hans. 2011. *The Sacredness of the Person: A New Genealogy of Human Rights*. Washington, DC: Georgetown University Press. Translated by Alex Skinner.

Joas, Hans, and Wolfgang Knobl. 2009. *Social Theory: Twenty Introductory Lectures*. Cambridge: Cambridge University Press.

Jacobson, Nora. 2012. *Dignity and Health*. Vanderbilt University Press.

Jacobson, Nora. 2007. "Dignity and Health: A Review." *Social Science & Medicine* 64 (2): 292–302.

Jylhä, Marja. 2009. "What Is Self-Rated Health and Why Does It Predict Mortality? Towards a Unified Conceptual Model." *Social Science & Medicine* 69 (3): 307–16.

Kahneman, Daniel. 2011. *Thinking, Fast and Slow*. Macmillan.

Kalleberg, Arne. 2009. "Precarious Work, Insecure Workers: Employment Relations in Transition." *American Sociological Review* 74: 1–22.

Kalleberg, Arne. 2018. *Precarious Lives: Job Insecurity and Well-Being in Rich Democracies*. Cambridge: Polity Press.

Kashima, Yoshihisa, Margaret Foddy, and Michael Platow. 2002. *Self and Identity: Personal, Social, and Symbolic*. Psychology Press.

Kasser, Tim. 2003. *The High Price of Materialism*. MIT Press.

Kiatpongsan, Sorapop, and Michael I. Norton. 2014. "How Much (More) Should CEOs Make? A Universal Desire for More Equal Pay." *Perspectives on Psychological Science* 9 (6): 587–93.

Killingsworth, Matthew A. 2021. "Experienced Well-Being Rises with Income, Even Above $75,000 per Year." *Proceedings of the National Academy of Sciences* 118 (4): e2016976118.

Killmister, Suzy. 2010. "Dignity: Not Such a Useless Concept." *Journal of Medical Ethics* 36 (3): 160–64.

King, Ryan D., and Brian D. Johnson. 2016. "A Punishing Look: Skin Tone and Afrocentric Features in the Halls of Justice." *American Journal of Sociology* 122 (1): 90–124.

Koskinen, Emmi, Melisa Stevanovic, and Anssi Peräkylä. 2011. "The Recognition and Interactional Management of Face Threats: Comparing Neurotypical Participants with Participants with Asperger's Syndrome." *Social Psychology Quarterly* 84: 132–54.

Kraus, M. W., I. N. Onyeador, N. M. Daumeyer, J. M. Rucker, and J. A. Richeson. 2019. "The Misperception of Racial Economic Inequality." *Perspectives on Psychological Science* 14 (6): 899–921.

Kuh, Diana, and Yoav Ben Shlomo, eds. 2004. *A Life Course Approach to Chronic Disease Epidemiology*. Oxford University Press.

Kwon, Hye Won. 2017. "The Sociology of Grit: Exploring Grit as a Sociological Variable and Its Potential Role in Social Stratification." *Sociology Compass* 11 (12): e12544.

Lakoff, Goerge, and Mark Johnson. 1999. *Philosophy in the Flesh: The Embodied Mind and Its Challenge to Western Thought*. New York: Basic Books.

Lakoff, George, and Mark Johnson. 2008. *Metaphors We Live By*. University of Chicago Press.

Lambert, Susan J., Julia R. Henly, and Jaeseung Kim. 2019. "Precarious Work Schedules as a Source of Economic Insecurity and Institutional Distrust." *RSF Journal of the Social Sciences* 5: 218–57.

Lamont, Michèle. 2000. *The Dignity of Working Men: Morality and the Boundaries of Gender, Race and Class*. Cambridge, MA: Harvard University Press.

Lamont, Michèle. 2017. "Prisms of Inequality: Moral Boundaries, Exclusion and Academic Evaluation." Prize Essay, Erasmus Prize, Amsterdam.

Lamont, Michèle. 2018. "Addressing Recognition Gaps: Destigmatization and the Reduction of Inequality." *American Sociological Review* 83: 419–44.

Lamont, Michèle. 2019. "From 'Having' to 'Being': Self-Worth and the Current Crisis of American Society." *British Journal of Sociology* 70: 660–707.

Lamont, Michèle, Graziella Moraes Silva, Jessica Welburn, Joshua Guetzkow, Nissim Mizrachi, Hanna Herzog, and Elisa Reis. 2016. *Getting Respect: Responding to Stigma and Discrimination in the United States, Brazil, and Israel.* Princeton University Press.

Lamont, Michèle, and Laurent Thévenot, eds. 2000. *Rethinking Comparative Cultural Sociology: Repertoires of Evaluation in France and the United States.* New York: Cambridge University Press.

Lareau, Annette. 2011. *Unequal Childhoods: Class, Race, and Family Life.* University of California Press.

Lawler, Edward J., Shane R. Thye, and Jeongkoo Yoon. 2015. *Order on the Edge of Chaos: Social Psychology and the Problem of Social Order.* New York: Cambridge University Press.

Lawrence, Elizabeth M. 2017. "Why Do College Graduates Behave More Healthfully Than Those Who Are Less Educated?" *Journal of Health and Social Behavior* 58 (3): 291–306.

Lee, Byungkyu, and Peter Bearman. 2020. "Political Isolation in America." *Network Science* 8 (3): 333–55.

Legewie, Joscha, and Thomas A. DiPrete. 2014. "The High School Environment and the Gender Gap in Science and Engineering." *Sociology of Education* 87 (4): 259–80.

Levy, Becca R., et al. 2009. "Age Stereotypes Held Earlier in Life Predict Cardiovascular Events in Later Life." *Psychological Science* 20 (3): 296–98.

Lichterman, Paul. 1995. "Beyond the Seesaw Model: Public Commitment in a Culture of Self-Fulfillment." *Sociological Theory* 13 (3): 275–300.

Lin, Nan. 2002. *Social Capital: A Theory of Social Structure and Action.* Cambridge University Press.

Lindemann, Gesa. 2015. "Human Dignity as a Structural Feature of Functional Differentiation—A Precondition for Modern Responsibilization." *Soziale Systeme* 19 (2): 235–58.

Link, Bruce G., and Jo Phelan. 1995. "Social Conditions as Fundamental Causes of Disease." *Journal of Health and Social Behavior* (extra issue): 80–94.

Lizardo, Omar. 2017. "Improving Cultural Analysis: Considering Personal Culture in Its Declarative and Nondeclarative Modes." *American Sociological Review* 82: 88–115.

Lucas, Kristen. 2015. "Workplace Dignity: Communicating Inherent, Earned, and Remediated Dignity." *Journal of Management Studies* 52 (5): 621–46.

Lucas, Samuel R. 2001. "Effectively Maintained Inequality: Education Transitions, Track Mobility, and Social Background Effects." *American Journal of Sociology* 106 (6): 1642–90.

Lucas, Samuel R. 2009. "Stratification Theory, Socioeconomic Background, and Educational Attainment: A Formal Analysis." *Rationality and Society* 21 (4): 459–511.

Luft, Aliza. 2020. "Theorizing Moral Cognition: Culture in Action, Situations, and Relationships." *Socius: Sociological Research for a Dynamic World* 6: 237802312091612. doi:10.1177/2378023120916125.

Luft, Aliza. 2022. "Dehumanization as Consequence, Not Cause, of Violence: Evidence from Rwanda." Working Paper, Department of Sociology, University of California—Los Angeles. Retrieved from SocArXiv on June 12, 2022.

Luhmann, Niklas. 1965. *Grundrechte als Institution*. Vol. 3. Berlin.

Lukes, Steven. 2008. *Moral Relativism*. New York: Picador.

Lupton, Deborah. 2016. "The Diverse Domains of Quantified Selves: Self-Tracking Modes and Dataveillance." *Economy and Society* 45 (1): 101–22.

Lutfey, Karen, and Jeremy Freese. 2005. "Toward Some Fundamentals of Fundamental Causality: Socioeconomic Status and Health in the Routine Clinic Visit for Diabetes." *American Journal of Sociology* 110 (5): 1326–72.

Macfarlane, Robert. 1996. *Landmarks*. New York: Penguin Books.

Macklin, Ruth. 2003. "Dignity Is a Useless Concept." *BMJ* 327 (7429): 1419–20.

Major, Brenda, John F. Dovidio, and Bruce G. Link, eds. 2018. *The Oxford Handbook of Stigma, Discrimination, and Health*. Oxford University Press.

Malpas, Jeff. 2007. "Human Dignity and Human Being." In *Perspectives on Human Dignity: A Conversation*, edited by Jeff Malpas and Norelle Lickiss, 19–26. New York: Springer.

Malpas, Jeff, and Norelle Lickiss. 2007. "Introduction to a Conversation." In *Perspectives on Human Dignity: A Conversation*, edited by Jeff Malpas and Norelle Lickiss, 1–8. New York: Springer.

Markovits, Daniel. 2019. *The Meritocracy Trap*. Penguin UK.

Markus, Hazel R., and Shinobu Kitayama. 1991. "Culture and the Self: Implications for Cognition, Emotion, and Motivation." *Psychological Review* 98 (2): 224.

Markus, Hazel, and Paula Nurius. 1986. "Possible Selves." *American Psychologist* 41 (9): 954.

Marmot, M. 2004. "Dignity and Inequality." *Lancet* 364: 1019–21.

Marmot, Michael. 2015. "The Health Gap: The Challenge of an Unequal World." *The Lancet* 386 (10011): 2442–44.

Martin, John Levi. 2001. "On the Limits of Sociological Theory." *Philosophy of the Social Sciences* 31: 187–223.

Martin, John Levi. 2003. "What Is Field Theory?" *American Journal of Sociology* 109 (1): 1–49.

Martin, John Levi. 2011. *The Explanation of Social Action*. New York: Oxford University Press.

Martin, John Levi, and Alessandra Lembo. 2020. "On the Other Side of Values." *American Journal of Sociology* 126: 52–98.

Massey, Douglas S., Jonathan Rothwell, and Thurston Domina. 2009. "The Changing Bases of Segregation in the United States." *Annals of the American Academy of Political and Social Science* 626 (1): 74–90.

Masten, Ann S., and Dante Cicchetti. 2010. "Developmental Cascades." *Development and Psychopathology* 22 (3): 491–95.

Masters, Ryan K., Bruce G. Link, and Jo C. Phelan. 2015. "Trends in Education Gradients of 'Preventable' Mortality: A Test of Fundamental Cause Theory." *Social Science & Medicine* 127: 19–28.

May, Todd. 2017. *A Fragile Life: Accepting Our Vulnerability*. University of Chicago Press.

Mayer, Emeran A. 2011. "Gut Feelings: The Emerging Biology of Gut–Brain Communication." *Nature Reviews Neuroscience* 12 (8): 453–66.

Mayer, Karl Ulrich. 2009. "New Directions in Life Course Research." *Annual Review of Sociology* 35: 413–33.

McAdams, Dan P. 2013a. "The Psychological Self as Actor, Agent, and Author." *Perspectives on Psychological Science* 8 (3): 272–95.

McAdams, Dan P. 2013b. *The Redemptive Self*. New York: Oxford University Press.

McCall, Leslie. 2013. *The Undeserving Rich: American Beliefs about Inequality, Opportunity, and Redistribution*. Cambridge University Press.

McCrudden, Christopher. 2013. "In Pursuit of Human Dignity: An Introduction to Current Debates." In *Understanding Human Dignity, Proceedings of the British Academy/Oxford University Press*, Forthcoming, U of Michigan Public Law Research Paper 309. Available at SSRN: https://ssrn.com/abstract=2218788

McLanahan, Sara S., and Erin L. Kelly. 2006. "The Feminization of Poverty." In *Handbook of the Sociology of Gender*, edited by Janet Saltzman Chafetz, 127–45. Boston: Springer.

McLeod, Jane D., Tim Hallett, and Kathryn J. Lively. 2015. "Beyond Three Faces: Toward an Integrated Social Psychology of Inequality." In *Advances in Group Processes*, Vol. 32, 1–29. Bingley, UK: Emerald Group Publishing Limited.

Mead, George Herbert, ed. 1934. *Mind, Self & Society from the Standpoint of a Social Behaviorist*. Chicago: University of Chicago Press.

Merton, Robert K. 1934. "Durkheim's Division of Labor in Society." *American Journal of Sociology* 40 (3): 319–28.

Metz, Thaddeus. 2014. "Dignity in the Ubuntu Tradition." In *Cambridge Handbook on Human Dignity*, edited by M. Düwell, J. Braarvig, R. Brownsword, and D. Mieth, 310–18. Cambridge: Cambridge University Press.

Mijs, Jonathan J. B. 2018. "Visualizing Belief in Meritocracy, 1930–2010." *Socius* 4: 1–2.

Mijs, Jonathan J. B. 2021. "The Paradox of Inequality: Income Inequality and Belief in Meritocracy Go Hand in Hand." *Socio-Economic Review* 19 (1): 7–35.

Miles, Andrew. 2015. "The (Re)genesis of Values: Examining the Importance of Values for Action." *American Sociological Review* 80: 680–704.

Miller, Sarah Clark. 2017. "Reconsidering Dignity Relationally." *Ethics and Social Welfare* 11: 108–21.

Mills, C. Wright. 1940. "Situated Actions and Vocabularies of Motive." *American Sociological Review* 5 (6): 904–13.

Mills, C. Wright, ed. 1959. *The Sociological Imagination*. New York: Oxford University Press.

Mirowsky, John. 2011. "Wage Slavery or Creative Work?" *Society and Mental Health* 1 (2): 73–88.

Mirowsky, John, and Catherine E. Ross. 1999. "Economic Hardship across the Life Course." *American Sociological Review* 64 (4): 548–69.

Mirowsky, John, and Catherine E. Ross. 2003. *Education, Social Status, and Health*. New York: Aldine de Gruyter.

Mirowsky, John, and Catherine E. Ross. 2005. "Education, Learned Effectiveness and Health." *London Review of Education* 3 (3): 205–20.

Mirowsky, John, and Catherine E. Ross. 2007. "Life Course Trajectories of Perceived Control and Their Relationship to Education." *American Journal of Sociology* 112 (5): 1339–82.

Mische, Ann. 2009. "Projects and Possibilities: Researching Futures in Action." *Sociological Forum* 24 (3).

Mischel, Walter, and Yuichi Shoda. 1995. "A Cognitive-Affective System Theory of Personality: Reconceptualizing Situations, Dispositions, Dynamics, and Invariance in Personality Structure." *Psychological Review* 102 (2): 246.

Misztal, Barbara A. 2013. "The Idea of Dignity: Its Modern Significance." *European Journal of Social Theory* 16 (1): 101–21. doi:10.1177/1368431012449237.

Monk Jr., Ellis P. 2020. "Linked Fate and Mental Health among African Americans." *Social Science & Medicine* 266: 113340.

Monk Jr., Ellis P. 2021. "Colorism and Physical Health: Evidence from a National Survey." *Journal of Health and Social Behavior* 62 (1): 37–52.

Monk Jr., Ellis P. 2022. "Inequality without Groups: Contemporary Theories of Categories, Intersectional Typicality, and the Disaggregation of Difference." *Sociological Theory* 40 (1): 3–27.

Montez, Jennifer Karas, et al. 2014. "Trends in Work–Family Context among US Women by Education Level, 1976 to 2011." *Population Research and Policy Review* 33 (5): 629–48.

Montez, Jennifer Karas, et al. 2018. "Does College Major Matter for Women's and Men's Health in Midlife? Examining the Horizontal Dimensions of Educational Attainment." *Social Science & Medicine* 198: 130–38.

Montez, Jennifer Karas, et al. 2019. "Educational Disparities in Adult Mortality across US States: How Do They Differ, and Have They Changed since the Mid-1980s?" *Demography* 56 (2): 621–44.

Montez, Jennifer Karas, Mark D. Hayward, and Anna Zajacova. 2021. "Trends in US Population Health: The Central Role of Policies, Politics, and Profits." *Journal of Health and Social Behavior* 62 (3): 286–301.

Morrison, Toni. 2019. *The Source of Self-Regard: Selected Essays, Speeches, and Meditations.* New York: Alfred A. Knopf.

Mueller, Anna S., et al. 2021. "The Social Roots of Suicide: Theorizing How the External Social World Matters to Suicide and Suicide Prevention." *Frontiers in Psychology* 12: 763.

Musick, Kelly, Ann Meier, and Sarah Flood. 2016. "How Parents Fare: Mothers' and Fathers' Subjective Well-Being in Time with Children." *American Sociological Review* 81 (5): 1069–95.

Neal, Mary. 2014. "Respect for Human Dignity as 'Substantive Basic Norm.'" *International Journal of Law in Context* 10: 26–46.

Neuhäuser, Christian, and Ralf Stoecker. 2014. "Human Dignity as Universal Nobility." In *Cambridge Handbook on Human Dignity*, edited by M. Düwell, J. Braarvig, R. Brownsword, and D. Mieth, 298–309. Cambridge: Cambridge University Press.

Nichols, Tom. 2017. *The Death of Expertise: The Campaign against Established Knowledge and Why It Matters.* Oxford University Press.

Noonan, Mary C., Freda B. Lynn, and Mark H. Walker. 2020. "Boxed In: Beliefs about the Compatibility and Likability of Mother-Occupation and Father-Occupation Role Combinations." *Socius* 6: 2378023120942449.

Norton, M., and D. Ariely. 2011. "Consensus on Building a Better America—One Wealth Quartile at a Time." *Perspectives on Psychological Science* 6: 9–12.

Oeur, Freeden. 2016. "Recognizing Dignity: Young Black Men Growing Up in an Era of Surveillance." *Socius* 2: 1–15.

O'Madagain, Cathal, and Michael Tomasello. 2022. "Shared Intentionality, Reason-Giving and the Evolution of Human Culture." *Philosophical Transactions of the Royal Society B* 377 (1843): 20200320.

Orol, Joshua Sassoon. 2019. "Aleph Pattern." *Poetry* 215 (1): 32–33.

Owens, Timothy J., Dawn T. Robinson, and Lynn Smith-Lovin. 2010. "Three Faces of Identity." *Annual Review of Sociology* 36 (1): 477–99.

Pager, Devah, and Hana Shepherd. 2008. "The Sociology of Discrimination: Racial Discrimination in Employment, Housing, Credit, and Consumer Markets." *Annual Review of Sociology* 34: 181.

Parish, Steven M. 2014. "Between Persons: How Concepts of the Person Make Moral Experience Possible." *Ethos* 42 (1): 31–50. doi:10.1111/etho.12037.

Pascoe, Elizabeth A., and Laura Smart Richman. 2009. "Perceived Discrimination and Health: A Meta-Analytic Review." *Psychological Bulletin* 135 (4): 531.

Paxton, Pamela, et al. 2011. *Nonrecursive Models: Endogeneity, Reciprocal Relationships, and Feedback Loops*. Vol. 168. Sage Publications.

Pearlin, Leonard I., and Alex Bierman. 2013. "Current Issues and Future Directions in Research into the Stress Process." In *Handbook of the Sociology of Mental Health*, 325–40. Dordrecht: Springer.

Pedulla, David S. 2018. "Emerging Frontiers in Audit Study Research: Mechanisms, Variation, and Representativeness." In *Audit Studies: Behind the Scenes with Theory, Method, and Nuance*, 179–95. Cham: Springer.

Pew Research Center. 2020. "Most Americans Say There Is Too Much Economic Inequality in the U.S., but Fewer Than Half Call It a Top Priority." Research Report, January 9.

Pew Research Center. 2021. "What Makes Life Meaningful? Views from 17 Advanced Economies." Research Report, November 18.

Phelps, Elizabeth A., and Joseph E. LeDoux. 2005. "Contributions of the Amygdala to Emotion Processing: From Animal Models to Human Behavior." *Neuron* 48 (2): 175–87.

Phillips, L. Taylor, and Brian S. Lowery. 2015. "The Hard-Knock Life? Whites Claim Hardships in Response to Racial Inequity." *Journal of Experimental Social Psychology* 61: 12–18.

Piliavin, Jane Allyn. 2008. "Altruism and Helping: The Evolution of a Field: The 2008 Cooley-Mead Presentation." *Social Psychology Quarterly* 72 (3): 209–25.

Pinker, Steven. 2008. "The Stupidity of Dignity." *New Republic* 28 (May): 28–31.

Pinker, Steven. 2018. *Enlightenment Now: The Case for Reason, Science, Humanism, and Progress*. Penguin UK.

Porpora, Douglas V. 2015. *Reconstructing Sociology: The Critical Realist Approach*. Cambridge University Press.

Post, Stephen G. 2022. *Dignity for Deeply Forgetful People: How Caregivers Can Meet the Challenges of Alzheimer's Disease*. JHU Press.

Pudrovska, Tetyana. 2013. "Job Authority and Breast Cancer." *Social Forces* 92 (1): 1–24.

Pudrovska, Tetyana, and Amelia Karraker. 2014. "Gender, Job Authority, and Depression." *Journal of Health and Social Behavior* 55 (4): 424–41.

Pugh, Allison J. 2012. "The Social Meanings of Dignity at Work." *Hedgehog Review* 14 (3): 30–39.

Quadlin, Natasha. 2018. "The Mark of a Woman's Record: Gender and Academic Performance in Hiring." *American Sociological Review* 83 (2): 331–60.

Quadlin, Natasha, and Brian Powell. 2022. *Who Should Pay? Higher Education, Responsibility, and the Public*. New York: Russell Sage Foundation.

Quillian, Lincoln, et al. 2017. "Meta-Analysis of Field Experiments Shows No Change in Racial Discrimination in Hiring over Time." *Proceedings of the National Academy of Sciences* 114 (41): 10870–75.

Ragin, Charles C. 1999. "Using Qualitative Comparative Analysis to Study Causal Complexity." *Health Services Research* 34 (5 Pt 2): 1225.

Rao, Aliya Hamid. 2021. "Gendered Interpretations of Job Loss and Subsequent Professional Pathways." *Gender & Society* 35 (6): 884–909.

Raphael, David Daiches. 1994. *Moral Philosophy.* New York: Oxford University Press.

Rawls, John. 1999. *A Theory of Justice.* Cambridge, MA: Belknap Press of Harvard University Press.

Rawls, John, and Sterling M. McMurrin, eds. 1987. "Liberty, Equality, and Law: Selected Tanner Lectures on Moral Philosophy." Salt Lake City: University of Utah Press.

Reardon, Sean F. 2011. "The Widening Academic Achievement Gap between the Rich and the Poor: New Evidence and Possible Explanations." *Whither Opportunity* 1 (1): 91–116.

Reardon, Sean F., Demetra Kalogrides, and Kenneth Shores. 2019. "The Geography of Racial/Ethnic Test Score Gaps." *American Journal of Sociology* 124 (4): 1164–221.

Resnik, Judith, and Julie Chi-hye Suk. 2003. "Adding Insult to Injury: Questioning the Role of Dignity in Conceptions of Sovereignty." *Stanford Law Review* 55: 1921–62.

Reynolds, Megan M. 2021. "Health Power Resources Theory: A Relational Approach to the Study of Health Inequalities." *Journal of Health and Social Behavior* 62 (4): 493–511.

Ricoeur, Paul. 1992. *Oneself as Another.* Translated by Kathleen Blamey. Chicago: University of Chicago Press.

Ridgeway, Cecilia L. 2009. "Framed before We Know It: How Gender Shapes Social Relations." *Gender & Society* 23 (2): 145–60.

Ridgeway, Cecilia L. 2011. *Framed by Gender: How Gender Inequality Persists in the Modern World.* New York: Oxford University Press.

Ridgeway, Cecilia L. 2014. "Why Status Matters for Inequality." *American Sociological Review* 79 (1): 1–16.

Ridgeway, Cecilia L. 2019. *Status: Why Is It Everywhere? Why Does It Matter?* Russell Sage Foundation.

Ridgeway, Cecilia L., and Shelley J. Correll. 2004. "Motherhood as a Status Characteristic." *Journal of Social Issues* 60: 683–700.

Riesman, David, Nathan Glazer, and Reuel Denney. 2020. *The Lonely Crowd.* Yale University Press.

Rinaldo, Rachel, and Jeffrey Guhin. 2019. "How and Why Interviews Work: Ethnographic Interviews and Meso-Level Public Culture." *Sociological Methods & Research* 51 (1): 34–67.

Robinson, Zandria Felice. 2016. "Intersectionality." In *Handbook of Contemporary Sociological Theory,* edited by Seth Abrutyn, 477–99. New York: Springer.

Rodriguez, Cristian G., et al. 2022. "Morbid Polarization: Exposure to COVID-19 and Partisan Disagreement about Pandemic Response." *Political Psychology* 43 (6): 1169–89.

Roscigno, Vincent J., Jill E. Yavorsky, and Natasha Quadlin. 2021. "Gendered Dignity at Work." *American Journal of Sociology* 127: 562–620.

Rosen, Michael. 2012. *Dignity: Its History and Meaning.* Cambridge, MA: Harvard University Press.

Rosenberg, Morris, et al. 1995. "Global Self-Esteem and Specific Self-Esteem: Different Concepts, Different Outcomes." *American Sociological Review* 60 (1): 141–56.

Rosling, Hans. 2018. *Factfulness: Ten Reasons We're Wrong about the World—And Why Things Are Better Than You Think*. New York: Flatiron Books.

Ross, Catherine E., Ryan K. Masters, and Robert A. Hummer. 2012. "Education and the Gender Gaps in Health and Mortality." *Demography* 49 (4): 1157–83.

Salzberg, Sharon. 2003. *Faith: Trusting Your Own Deepest Experience*. New York: Penguin Books.

Sanchez, Mari, Michèle Lamont, and Shira Zilberstein. 2022. "How American College Students Understand Social Resilience and Navigate towards the Future during Covid and the Movement for Racial Justice." *Social Science & Medicine* 301: 114890. doi:10.1016/j.socscimed.2022.114890.

Sandel, Michael J. 2020. *The Tyranny of Merit: What's Become of the Common Good?* New York: Farrar, Straus, and Giroux.

Sassler, Sharon, et al. 2017. "The Missing Women in STEM? Assessing Gender Differentials in the Factors Associated with Transition to First Jobs." *Social Science Research* 63: 192–208.

Sauder, Michael, and Wendy Nelson Espeland. 2009. "The Discipline of Rankings: Tight Coupling and Organizational Change." *American Sociological Review* 74 (1): 63–82.

Sayer, Andrew. 2007. "Dignity at Work: Broadening the Agenda." *Organization* 14 (4): 565–81.

Sayer, Andrew. 2011. *Why Things Matter to People: Social Science, Values, and Ethical Life*. Cambridge: Cambridge University Press.

Sayer, Liana C., Vicki A. Freedman, and Suzanne M. Bianchi. 2016. "Gender, Time Use, and Aging." In *Handbook of Aging and the Social Sciences*, 163–80. Academic Press.

Schieman, Scott, and Jonathan Koltai. 2017. "Discovering Pockets of Complexity: Socioeconomic Status, Stress Exposure, and the Nuances of the Health Gradient." *Social Science Research* 63: 1–18.

Schilke, Oliver, Martin Reimann, and Karen S. Cook. 2021. "Trust in Social Relations." *Annual Review of Sociology* 47: 239–59.

Schneider, Daniel, and Kristen Harknett. 2019. "Consequences of Routine Work-Schedule Instability for Worker Health and Well-Being." *American Sociological Review* 84 (1): 82–114.

Schnittker, Jason. 2013. "Social Structure and Personality." In *Handbook of Social Psychology*, edited by John DeLamater and Amanda Ward, 89–115. New York: Springer.

Schnittker, Jason, and Jane D. McLeod. 2005. "The Social Psychology of Health Disparities." *Annual Review of Sociology* 31: 75–103.

Schudde, Lauren, and Raymond Stanley Brown. 2019. "Understanding Variation in Estimates of Diversionary Effects of Community College Entrance: A Systematic Review and Meta-Analysis." *Sociology of Education* 92 (3): 247–68.

Schur, Michael. 2022. *How to Be Perfect: The Correct Answer to Every Moral Question*. New York: Simon & Schuster.

Schwalbe, Michael, et al. 2000. "Generic Processes in the Reproduction of Inequality: An Interactionist Analysis." *Social Forces* 79 (2): 419–52.

Schwartz, Shalom H. 2017. "The Refined Theory of Basic Values." In *Values and Behavior*, edited by S. Roccas and L. Sagiv, 51–72. Cham, Switzerland: Springer.

Schwartz, Shalom H., and Wolfgang Bilsky. 1987. "Toward a Psychological Structure of Human Values." *Journal of Personality and Social Psychology* 53: 550–62.

Scott, James C. 1976. *The Moral Economy of the Peasant*. New Haven, CT: Yale University Press.

Scruggs, Lyle, and Thomas J. Hayes. 2017. "The Influence of Inequality on Welfare Generosity: Evidence from the US States." *Politics & Society* 45 (1): 35–66.

Seamster, Louise, and Raphaël Charron-Chénier. 2017. "Predatory Inclusion and Education Debt: Rethinking the Racial Wealth Gap." *Social Currents* 4 (3): 199–207.

Seamster, Louise, and Victor Ray. 2018. "Against Teleology in the Study of Race: Toward the Abolition of the Progress Paradigm." *Sociological Theory* 36 (4): 315–42.

Sehgal, Neil Jay, et al. 2022. "The Association between COVID-19 Mortality and the County-Level Partisan Divide in the United States: Study Examines the Association between COVID-19 Mortality and County-Level Political Party Affiliation." *Health Affairs* 41 (6): 853–63.

Seligman, Hilary K., and Seth A. Berkowitz. 2019. "Aligning Programs and Policies to Support Food Security and Public Health Goals in the United States." *Annual Review of Public Health* 40: 319.

Sen, Amartya. 2000. "A Decade of Human Development." *Journal of Human Development* 1 (1): 17–23.

Sennett, Richard. 2003. *Respect: The Formation of Character in a World of Inequalities.* New York: Alfred K. Knopf.

Sennett, Richard, and Jonathan Cobb. [1972] 1993. *The Hidden Injuries of Class.* New York: W. W. Norton.

Sensen, Oliver. 2011. "Human Dignity in Historical Perspective: The Contemporary and Traditional Paradigms." *European Journal of Political Theory* 10 (1): 71–91.

Sewell Jr., William H. 1992. "A Theory of Structure: Duality, Agency, and Transformation." *American Journal of Sociology* 98 (1): 1–29.

Shanahan, Michael J., and Kathryn E. Hood. 2000. "Adolescents in Changing Social Structures: Bounded Agency in Life Course Perspective." In *Negotiating Adolescence in Times of Social Change,* edited by Rainer Silbereisen and Elizabeth Crockett, 123–34. Cambridge, UK: Cambridge University Press.

Shelton, Suzanne H. 1990. "Developing the Construct of General Self-Efficacy." *Psychological Reports* 66 (3): 987–94.

Shilling, Chris, and Philip A. Mellor. 2022. "Social Character, Interdependence, and the Dualities of Other-Directedness." *British Journal of Sociology* 73 (1): 125–38.

Shuey, Kim M., and Andrea E. Willson. 2014. "Economic Hardship in Childhood and Adult Health Trajectories: An Alternative Approach to Investigating Life-Course Processes." *Advances in Life Course Research* 22: 49–61.

shuster, stef m. 2016. "Uncertain Expertise and the Limitations of Clinical Guidelines in Transgender Healthcare." *Journal of Health and Social Behavior* 57 (3): 319–32.

shuster, stef m. 2022. *Trans Medicine: The Emergence and Practice of Treating Gender.* New York: New York University Press.

Shweder, Richard A. 1991. *Thinking through Cultures: Expeditions in Cultural Psychology.* Cambridge, MA: Harvard University Press.

Siegrist, Johannes, and Michael Marmot. 2004. "Health Inequalities and the Psychosocial Environment—Two Scientific Challenges." *Social Science & Medicine* 58 (8): 1463–73.

Silva, Jennifer M. 2013. *Coming Up Short: Working-Class Adulthood in an Age of Uncertainty.* Oxford: Oxford University Press.

Simmel, Georg. 1950. *The Sociology of Georg Simmel.* New York: Free Press.

Simmel, Georg. 2012. "Group Expansion and the Development of Individuality." In *Classic Sociological Theory,* edited by Craig Calhoun, Joseph Gerteis, James Moody, Steven Pfaff, and Indermohan Virk, 366–81. Malden, MA: Wiley-Blackwell.

Skorpen, Frode, Arne Rehnsfeldt, and Arlene Arstad Thorsen. 2015. "The Significance of Small Things for Dignity in Psychiatric Care." *Nursing Ethics* 22 (7): 754–64.

Smith, Christian. 2003. *Moral, Believing Animals*. Chicago: University of Chicago Press.

Smith, Christian. 2009. *What Is a Person?* Chicago: University of Chicago Press.

Smith, Zadie. 2020. *Intimations: Six Essays*. New York: Penguin Books.

Snow, David A., and Leon Anderson. 1987. "Identity Work among the Homeless: The Verbal Construction and Avowal of Personal Identities." *American Journal of Sociology* 92 (6): 1336–71.

Starmans, Christina, Mark Sheskin, and Paul Bloom. 2017. "Why People Prefer Unequal Societies." *Nature Human Behaviour* 1 (4): 1–7.

Steinmetz, George. 2014. "The Sociology of Empires, Colonies, and Postcolonialism." *Annual Review of Sociology* 40: 77–103.

Stets, Jan E., and Peter J. Burke. 2000. "Identity Theory and Social Identity Theory." *Social Psychology Quarterly* 63 (3): 224–37.

Sulmasy, Daniel P. 2007. "Human Dignity and Human Worth." In *Perspectives on Human Dignity: A Conversation*, edited by Jeff Malpas and Norelle Lickiss, 9–18. New York: Springer.

Sulmasy, Daniel P. 2013. "The Varieties of Human Dignity: A Logical and Conceptual Analysis." *Medicine, Health Care and Philosophy* 16: 937–44.

Swidler, Ann. 1986. "Culture in Action: Symbols and Strategies." *American Sociological Review* 51 (2): 273–86.

Swidler, Ann. 2001. *Talk of Love: How Culture Matters*. Chicago: University of Chicago Press.

Taylor, Charles, ed. 1991. *The Ethics of Authenticity*. Cambridge, MA: Harvard University Press.

Taylor, Charles. 1992. *Sources of the Self: The Making of the Modern Identity*. Harvard University Press.

Taylor, Charles. 1994. "Reply to Commentators." *Philosophy and Phenomenological Research* 54 (1): 203–13.

Tesser, Abraham, et al. 2000. "Confluence of Self-Esteem Regulation Mechanisms: On Integrating the Self-Zoo." *Personality and Social Psychology Bulletin* 26 (12): 1476–89.

Thaler, Richard M. 2016. *Misbehaving*. New York: W. W. Norton.

Thoits, Peggy A. 1983. "Multiple Identities and Psychological Well-Being: A Reformulation and Test of the Social Isolation Hypothesis." *American Sociological Review* 48 (2): 174–87.

Thomas, W. I., and Dorothy Swain Thomas. 1928. *The Child in America: Behavior Problems and Programs*. New York: Knopf.

Tilcsik, András. 2021. "Statistical Discrimination and the Rationalization of Stereotypes." *American Sociological Review* 86 (1): 93–122.

Timmermans, Stefan, and Marc Berg. 2010. *The Gold Standard: The Challenge of Evidence-Based Medicine*. Temple University Press.

Tomaskovic-Devey, Don, and Sheryl Skaggs. 2002. "Sex Segregation, Labor Process Organization, and Gender Earnings Inequality." *American Journal of Sociology* 108 (1): 102–28.

Turner, Jonathan H. 1987. "Toward a Sociological Theory of Motivation." *American Journal of Sociology* 52: 15–27.

Turner, Ralph H. 1976. "The Real Self: From Institution to Impulse." *American Journal of Sociology* 84: 1–23.

Turner, Ralph H. 1978. "The Role and the Person." *American Journal of Sociology* 84 (1): 1–23.

Turner, Ralph H., and Jerald Schutte. 1981. "The True Self Method for Studying the Self-Conception." *Symbolic Interaction* 4 (1): 1–20.

Tversky, Amos, and Daniel Kahneman. 1974. "Judgment under Uncertainty: Heuristics and Biases: Biases in Judgments Reveal Some Heuristics of Thinking under Uncertainty." *Science* 185 (4157): 1124–31.

Upenieks, Laura. 2022. "Perceptions of Dignity, Attachment to God, and Mental Health in a National US Sample." *Journal of Religion and Health* 61 (5): 1–22.

Vaisey, Stephen. 2009. "Motivation and Justification: A Dual-Process Model of Culture in Action." *American Journal of Sociology* 114 (6): 1675–715.

Van Hook, Jennifer, and Jennifer E. Glick. 2007. "Immigration and Living Arrangements: Moving beyond Economic Need versus Acculturation." *Demography* 44 (2): 225–49.

Van Hook, Jennifer, and Jennifer E. Glick. 2020. "Spanning Borders, Cultures, and Generations: A Decade of Research on Immigrant Families." *Journal of Marriage and Family* 82 (1): 224–43.

Verdery, Ashton M., et al. 2020. "Tracking the Reach of COVID-19 Kin Loss with a Bereavement Multiplier Applied to the United States." *Proceedings of the National Academy of Sciences* 117 (30): 17695–701.

Villalonga-Olives, Ester, and Ichiro Kawachi. 2017. "The Dark Side of Social Capital: A Systematic Review of the Negative Health Effects of Social Capital." *Social Science & Medicine* 194: 105–27.

Von Scheve, Christian. 2012. "Emotion Regulation and Emotion Work: Two Sides of the Same Coin?" *Frontiers in Psychology* 3: 496.

Wacquant, Loïc. 2014. "Putting Habitus in Its Place: Rejoinder to the Symposium." *Body & Society* 20 (2): 118–39.

Waldron, Jeremy. 2009. "Dignity, Rank, and Rights: The 2009 Tanner Lectures at UC Berkeley." NYU School of Law, Public Law Research Paper 09–50.

Waldron, Jeremy. 2015. *Dignity, Rank, & Rights*. New York: Oxford.

Waters, Mary C., and Philip Kasinitz. 2010. "Discrimination, Race Relations, and the Second Generation." *Social Research: An International Quarterly* 77 (1): 101–32.

Watkins-Hayes, Celeste. 2019. *Remaking a Life*. University of California Press.

Watkins-Hayes, Celeste, LaShawnDa Pittman-Gay, and Jean Beaman. 2012. "'Dying from' to 'Living with': Framing Institutions and the Coping Processes of African American Women Living with HIV/AIDS." *Social Science & Medicine* 74: 2028–36.

Weber, Max. 1958. *The Protestant Ethic and the Spirit of Capitalism*, translated by Talcott Parsons. New York: Scribner.

Weber, Max. 1981. *From Max Weber: Essays in Sociology*, edited by Hans H. Gerth and C. Wright Mills. New York: Oxford University Press.

Weinberger, Daniel M., et al. 2020. "Estimation of Excess Deaths Associated with the COVID-19 Pandemic in the United States, March to May 2020." *JAMA Internal Medicine* 180 (10): 1336–44.

Weinrib, Jacob. 2016. *Dimensions of Dignity: The Theory and Practice of Modern Constitutional Law*. New York: Cambridge University Press.

Wherry, Frederick F., Kristin S. Seefeldt, and Anthony S. Alvarez. 2019. *Credit Where It's Due: Rethinking Financial Citizenship*. Russell Sage Foundation.

White, Harrison. 1992. *Identity and Control: A Structural Theory of Social Action.* Princeton, NJ: Princeton University Press.

Wilcoxson, Anna, and Kelly Moore. 2020. "Dignity Strategies in a Neoliberal Workfare Kitchen Training Program." *Sociological Inquiry* 90 (1): 30–51.

Wilkerson, Isabel. 2020. *Caste: The Origins of Our Discontents.* New York: Random House.

Williams, Christine L. 2021. "Life Support: The Problems of Working for a Living." *American Sociological Review* 86: 191–200.

Williams, David R. 2018. "Stress and the Mental Health of Populations of Color: Advancing Our Understanding of Race-Related Stressors." *Journal of Health and Social Behavior* 59 (4): 466–85.

Williams, D. R., and S. A. Mohammed. 2013. "Racism and Health I: Pathways and Scientific Evidence." *American Behavioral Scientist* 57 (8): 1152–73.

Wilson, William Julius. 2012. *The Truly Disadvantaged: The Inner City, the Underclass, and Public Policy.* University of Chicago Press.

Wingfield, Adia Harvey. 2010. "Are Some Emotions Marked 'Whites Only'? Racialized Feeling Rules in Professional Workplaces." *Social Problems* 57 (2): 251–68.

Wingfield, Adia Harvey. 2019. *Flatlining: Race, Work, and Health Care in the New Economy.* University of California Press.

Wrong, Dennis H. 1961. "The Oversocialized Conception of Man in Modern Sociology." *American Sociological Review* 26: 183–93.

Xiao, Jinnan, et al. 2019. "Effects of Dignity Therapy on Dignity, Psychological Well-Being, and Quality of Life among Palliative Care Cancer Patients: A Systematic Review and Meta-Analysis." *Psycho-Oncology* 28 (9): 1791–802.

Yang, Song, Brandon A. Jackson, and Anna Zajicek. 2021. "A Changing Landscape? An Intersectional Analysis of Race and Gender Disparity in Access to Social Capital." *Sociological Spectrum* 41 (1): 80–95.

Zajacova, Anna, et al. 2020. "The Relationship between Education and Pain among Adults Aged 30–49 in the United States." *Journal of Pain* 21 (11–12): 1270–80.

Zajacova, Anna, Hanna Grol-Prokopczyk, and Zachary Zimmer. 2021. "Pain Trends among American Adults, 2002–2018: Patterns, Disparities, and Correlates." *Demography* 58 (2): 711–38.

Zajacova, Anna, and Elizabeth M. Lawrence. 2018. "The Relationship between Education and Health: Reducing Disparities through a Contextual Approach." *Annual Review of Public Health* 39: 273–89.

Zajacova, Anna, and Elizabeth Lawrence. 2021. "Postsecondary Educational Attainment and Health among Younger US Adults in the 'College-for-All' Era." *Socius* 7: 23780231211021197.

Zelizer, Viviana A. 1979. *Morals & Markets: The Development of Life Insurance in the United States.* New Brunswick, NJ: Transaction Books.

Zelizer, Viviana. 1994. *The Social Meaning of Money.* Princeton, NJ: Princeton University Press.

Zelizer, Viviana. 2010. *Economic Lives.* Princeton, NJ: Princeton University Press.

Zewde, Naomi, and Christopher Wimer. 2019. "Antipoverty Impact of Medicaid Growing with State Expansions Over Time." *Health Affairs* 38 (1): 132–38.

# Index